# by Jane Fonda

Photographs by Harry Langdon

# JANE FONDA'S NEW WORKOUT & WEIGHT-LOSS PROGRAMME

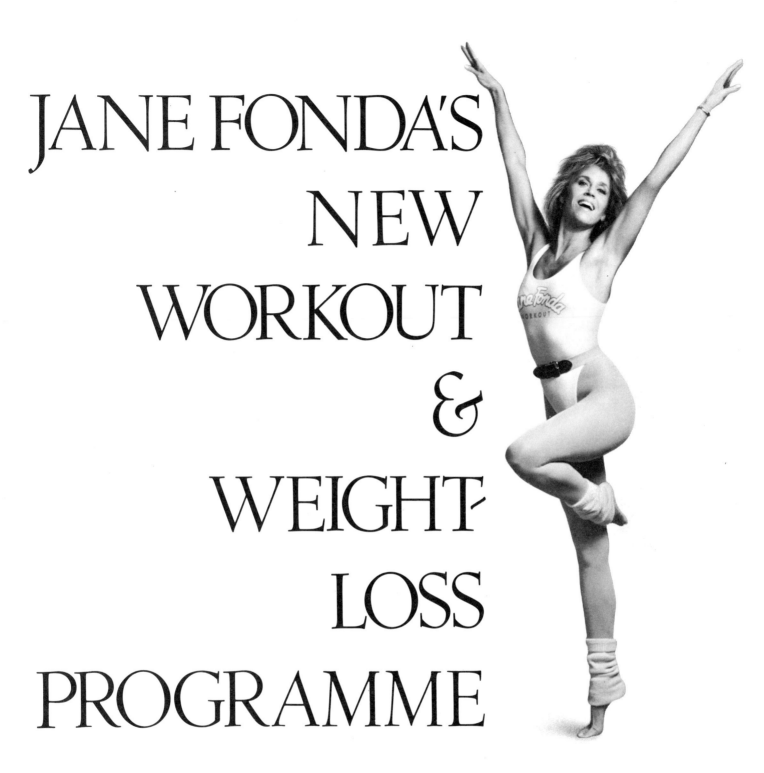

VIKING

VIKING
Penguin Books Ltd, Harmondsworth, Middlesex, England
Viking Penguin Inc., 40 West 23rd Street, New York, New York 10010, U.S.A.
Penguin Books Australia Ltd, Ringwood, Victoria, Australia
Penguin Books Canada Limited, 2801 John Street, Markham, Ontario, Canada L3R 1B4
Penguin Books (N.Z.) Ltd, 182–190 Wairau Road, Auckland 10, New Zealand

First published in the U.S.A. by Simon & Schuster, a division
of Simon & Schuster, Inc. 1986
First published in Great Britain by Viking 1987

Small portions of this work appeared in *Jane Fonda's Workout Book*,
copyright © 1981 by The Workout, Inc.

The recipe for Tomato Salad Dressing on page 59 is adapted from *Diet for Life*, by Francine Prince.
Copyright © 1981 by Francine Prince. Reprinted by permission of Simon and Schuster, Inc.
   The recipes for Cottage Cream on page 55 and for Tomato-Herb Dressing on page 60 are reprinted from
*Jane Brody's Good Food Book* by permission of the author and W. W. Norton and Company, Inc. Copyright
© 1985 by Jane E. Brody.
   The excerpt from *Bulimia: The Binge Purge Compulsion* by Janice M. Cauwels, copyright © 1983 by
Janice M. Cauwels, is reprinted by permission of Doubleday & Company, Inc.

Printed in Great Britain by
Butler & Tanner Ltd
Frome and London

*British Library Cataloguing in Publication Data available*
ISBN 0–670–81593–4

# ACKNOWLEDGMENTS

I want to especially thank my assistant, Debi Karolewski, without whose administrative skills and dogged humor my life would be a lot less pleasant and ordered.

In a brief lapse of sanity, Debi offered to add to her already overloaded workday the task of putting this book into our office computer—"a good way to learn the technology," she said.

Throughout the numerous rewrites and revisions and notwithstanding the day she was unable to retrieve an entire chapter from the bowels of the machine, it was Debi, sleeping in the office and working weekends, who made it possible for me to meet my deadline. I doubt that she would ever do it again.

In addition to Debi, my friend and cowriter on *Women Coming of Age,* Mignon McCarthy, gave me invaluable input and editorial assistance.

I am grateful for the expertise of Dr. James Garrick, director of the Center for Sports Medicine at St. Francis Memorial Hospital in San Francisco; Donna Gillien, the Center's director of research; Jeffrey Bland, Ph.D., director of the Linus Pauling Laboratory for Nutritional Research; and Dr. Michael Strober, director of the Teenage Eating Disorders Program at the U.C.L.A. Neuropsychiatric Institute.

As always, Harry Langdon and his staff are a pleasure to work with.

Thanks to my editor, Fred Hills; the book's designer, Eve Metz; my copy editor, Leslie Ellen; and photo editor, Vincent Virga. This is our third book together and they continue to make it an almost painless experience.

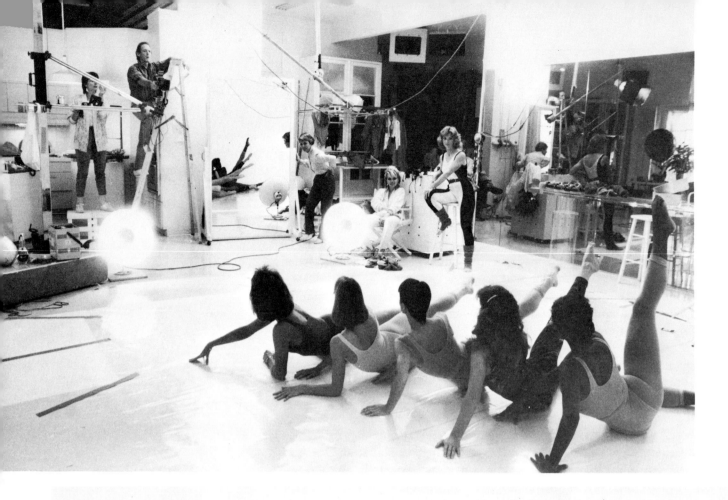

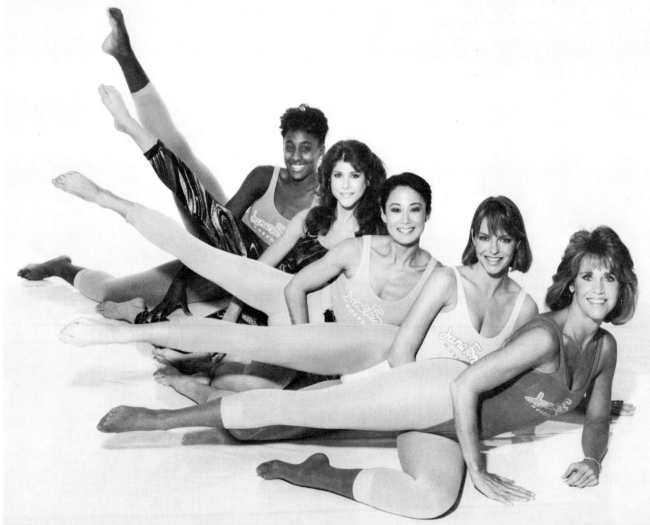

# CONTENTS

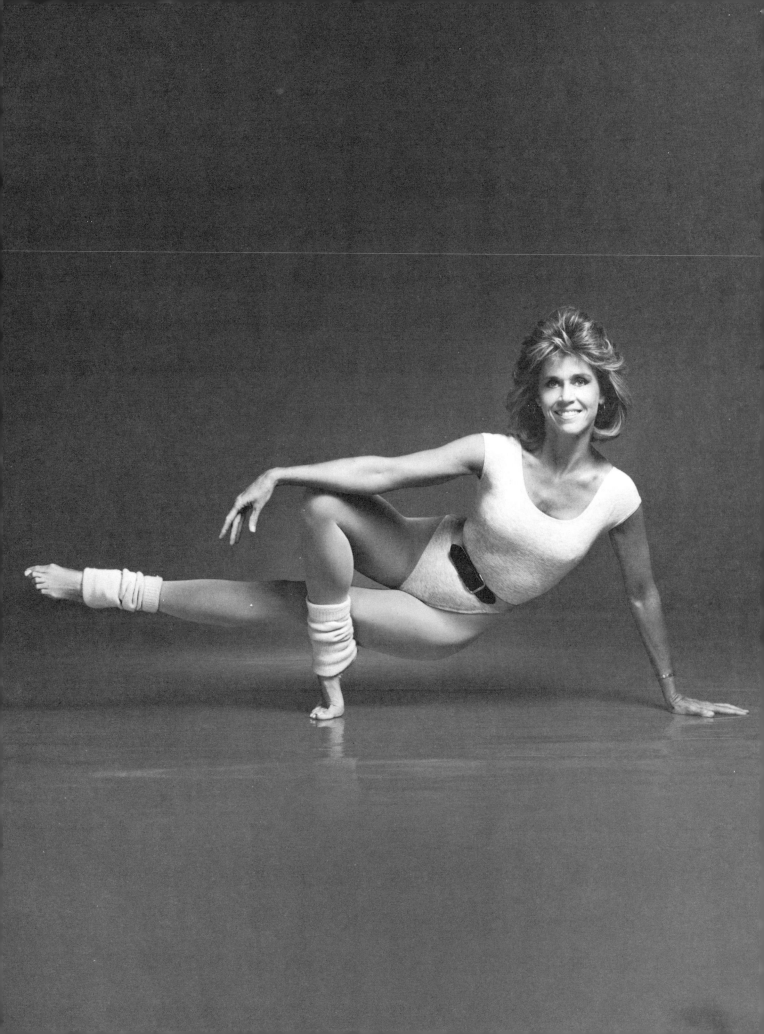

# INTRODUCTION

When someone first suggested to me that I create a diet to accompany the Workout, I reacted with skepticism. I am profoundly distressed by the deep and continuing preoccupation with weight in our society, and it seems to me that many of today's popular diets only perpetuate this obsession with thinness. But, finally, it was the very fact that so many of these diets are concerned only with shedding pounds, sometimes too quickly and sometimes dangerously, that made me feel that a safe, new weight-loss component to the Workout program was in fact needed, and that such a diet could be of considerable value to the many women who have asked me over the years for advice about dieting. I think this new Workout Weight-Loss Program fills a need and will help you to achieve safe and effective weight loss, while encouraging you to adopt a new goal for your body: vigorous health.

Working in close consultation with nutritionists and exercise physiologists, I have developed what I consider a "state of the art" diet and exercise program. The new exercise program is geared to burn calories and tone muscles faster, more effectively, and more efficiently than ever, without leaving you gasping for breath. In fact, the latest research shows that you actually burn fat more effectively if you don't become breathless while exercising. The diet is based on the low-fat, high-fiber, high–complex-carbohydrate diet that I began to develop in my first Workout book and that is now being recognized by the American Heart Association and others as the best, safest, and most healthful diet. It's a "free-choice" diet: it allows you a wide range of foods to select from and also allows you to adapt your own recipes and still stay within its guidelines. A diet can only be successful if you stick with it, and the flexibility of my free-choice diet makes it a nutritional program you can live with, without all the liabilities and counterproductivity of the standard quick-weight-loss, quick-regain diets.

In the first chapters I lay out the basics of nutrition, the springboard to a lifelong way of eating whether you are concerned about losing weight, gaining weight, or just staying where you are.

Then I present the new diet component of the Workout Weight-Loss Program, followed by the exercise component, which explains—in a way that I hope will motivate you—why exercise is an essential ingredient in shedding fat.

Next I integrate all the information that has become available to me into a section on how to exercise, how to get started, and how to choose a program; and, finally, the New Workout itself is demonstrated by four of my Workout teachers. (In a few instances where the basics remain un-

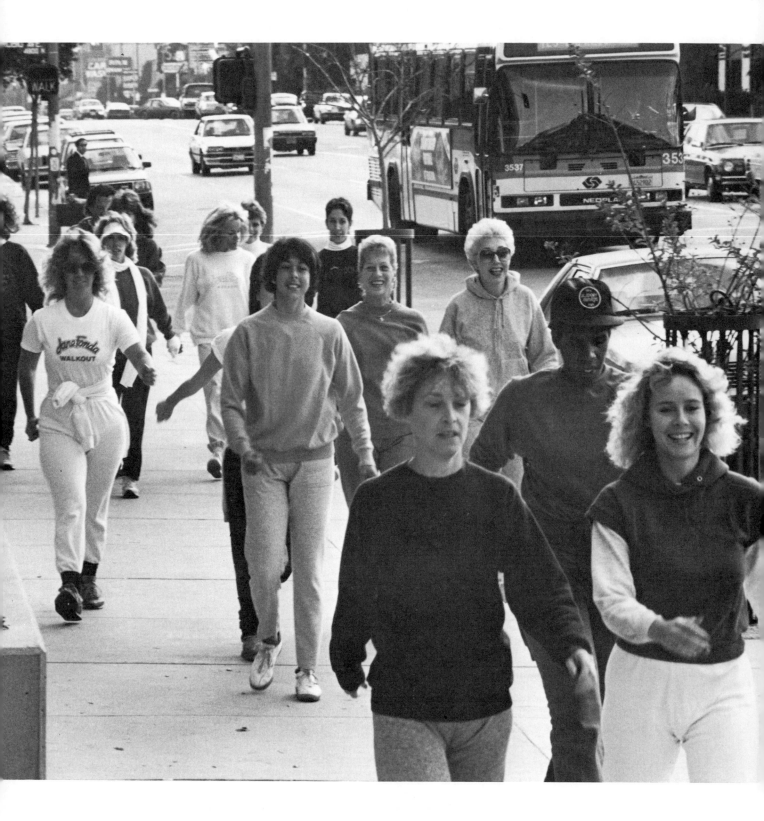

changed, I have drawn freely from the discussion in my first *Workout Book*.)

In these pages, I hope to encourage a more balanced approach to the whole issue of body weight and body image. I know firsthand the toll taken on our health and on our perception of ourselves by the obsessive approach. Such anxiety women suffer—over a little bulge in the belly or dimple in the thigh. When women who actually look malnourished voice these concerns —and we've all heard them do so—we're witnessing a sometimes tragic cultural phenomenon. The implication is that there is nothing worthy about us except the flatness and tautness of our bodies—as though these are the yardsticks against which our characters and lovableness are measured.

Since almost none of us are able to live up to these internalized, unrealistic standards, we hate ourselves and feel guilty and depressed. If only we were more disciplined, more determined, we think, we could be really thin and people would like us more. I devoted many pages in my first *Workout Book* to a discussion of how my own striving for skinniness—the diuretics, the bulimia, the starvation diets—had played havoc with my mind and body. I have always made a point of stressing that the goal of exercising and becoming fit is not to form yourself to the contours of some "fashionable" mold, not to look like someone else, but to make your own body as vibrant and healthy as it can be, to affirm your own uniqueness, to feel you can have a little control over your physical self in a positive way, and to overcome the alienation from our bodies that many of us feel.

This is what the Workout has done for me. Together with all that I've learned about healthy eating and safe and effective weight loss, the Workout has enabled me to be less frantic about being thin. It's helped me to be more relaxed, less compulsive about weight, while giving me the tools to maintain a *reasonable* weight—healthfully. For me, this is about 125 pounds, about ten pounds more than what I used to think I *should* weigh. In those days of compulsive eating and compulsive dieting, my body was always fighting me, as though trying to tell me that my goal wasn't appropriate for my body. Now I think I look better and I know I feel better than I ever did in my days of chronic dieting.

I know that it's extremely difficult to overcome a lifetime of cultural conditioning. There will be women who will exercise compulsively, as they eat (or refuse to eat) compulsively, in order to be thinner than they should be. But I do believe that for most of us, knowledge about nutrition and rational (not excessive) exercise can help us to like ourselves the way we are supposed to be, not the way fashion tells us we should be. Helping you achieve this approach to diet and exercise as a route to health—not as a means of getting thinner than you should be—is my goal.

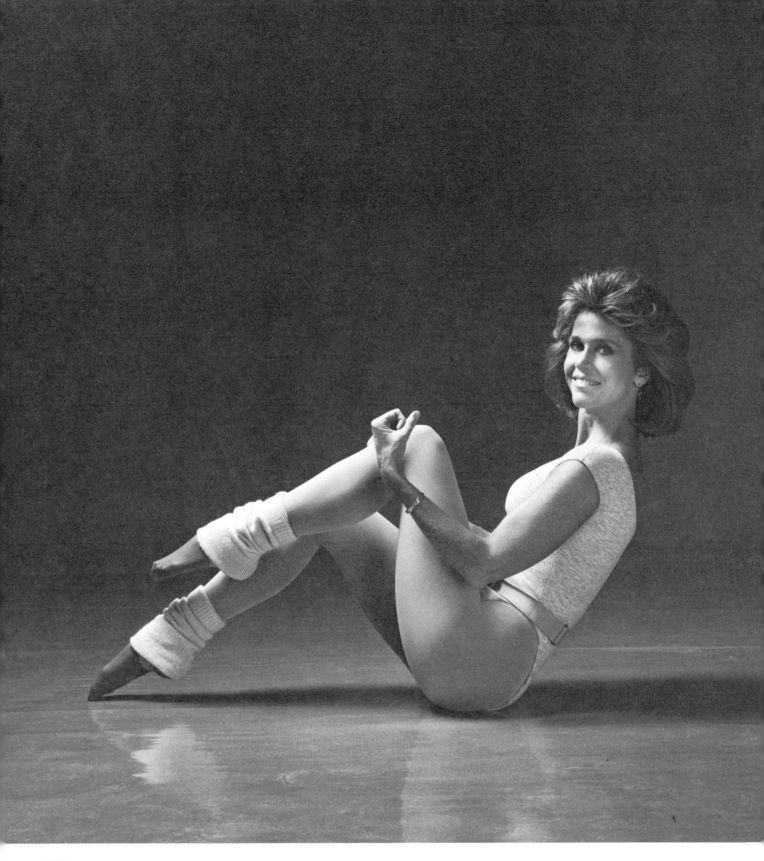

# I · EATING RIGHT

# THE SET-POINT THEORY: WHY FAD DIETS DON'T WORK

All women in our culture are subject to the pressure to be thin—an inordinate number of us begin stressful, long-standing patterns of undereating as a result. To a frightening degree, women's sense of self-esteem, power, control, and personal success derives from this ability to undereat—unlike men who gain their sense of acceptance, assertiveness, and confidence through competitive sports, corporate "gamesmanship," and other such opportunities in the public arena. The psychological and physical impact of this on women is serious. It damages their sense of self-worth and encourages destructive eating disorders such as anorexia and bulimia. This obsession with being thin also makes fad diets a way of life for many women.

There's probably not one of us who hasn't tried losing weight fast, *too fast,* through fad diets, fasting, overly restricting our caloric intake, and other such attempts at starving ourselves into thinness. There are two main problems with these all-too-common approaches to losing weight, however. First, they seriously jeopardize our health. And second, such dieting efforts are fundamentally counterproductive. Ultimately, they don't work.

- We lose fat, yes, but also a large measure of muscle.
- We unintentionally lower our metabolism.
- We set the stage for gaining fat increasingly faster in the future when we come off the diet, and thereby get caught up in perpetual dieting.
- We receive inadequate nutrients in imbalanced combinations.
- We tax the entire body.

Prolonged fasting, for instance, causes important electrolytes like sodium, calcium, magnesium, and phosphate to be excreted. Weakness and fainting can occur due to dehydration and a reduction in the volume of blood. Congestive heart failure and even death have been reported in cases of fasting and extremely low caloric intake.

Fasting and very low calorie diets (diets below 500 calories) cause a loss of nitrogen and potassium in the body, a loss which is believed to trigger a mechanism in the body that causes us to hold on to our fat stores and to turn to muscle protein for energy instead. Scientists have speculated that within each of us is a unique "set-point mechanism" that regulates the amount of fat we carry. It's believed to be a survival mechanism of our species, a way of stocking up for times of famine and emergency. If the body perceives that it's starving, as it rightly does if we are *always* on a diet or if we suddenly *crash*-diet or *fast,* the set point is thought to kick into action, causing the body to keep a tenacious grip on its fat supply. In order to replenish itself, the body will first cause you to *crave food*—most commonly fuel-dense, high-caloried sugars and fats. If you successfully resist these cravings, the body's next line of defense will be to react by *slowing down the metabolism* in order to conserve calories. In the face of food deprivation, the body holds on to its fat tissue for dear life.

Given all this, you should immediately rule out such approaches to weight loss. No system based on severe food deprivation is a wise way to lose weight. Even on a total fast, because you're losing muscle and altering your metabolism, you'll actually be losing *less* weight in the end than if you ate 1000–1200 calories of protein- and carbohydrate-rich foods every day, combined with exercise. Fad diets that have you eating one or two of the same foods over long periods of time deplete you of essential nutrients and result in the wasting away of muscles too. There is no scientific validity to these diets. Weight lost on high-fat, high-protein diets like the Atkins Diet is primarily water loss, and even that water is lost largely during the first few weeks. This weight is quickly gained back.

# THE BULIMIA CRISIS

For some women, chronically depriving themselves of food leads to one of two extreme forms of self-starvation: anorexia or bulimia. Bulimia is the severe eating disorder which I became acquainted with early on, in my teenage years.

As a little girl, I was healthily plump. But even that young, I had so internalized the cultural obsession with thinness that I was self-conscious about my roundness. I remember my older half-sister having written on the cover of her school notebook the title of a popular song back then: "June is busting out all over." When I saw the words, I thought they said, "*Jane* is busting out all over," and I was mortified. I was so conditioned to think of myself as fat that later, when I lost that childhood plumpness, when I became really thin, too thin, I could never convince myself that I was thin enough.

It was during my high school years, at boarding school, that I first learned about eating and throwing up. When my roommate told me about it, I thought to myself, "Aha! Here's a way to have my cake and *not* eat it too!" We could indulge our eating compulsions without having to face the consequences of getting fat. It gave us a heady sense of being in control. We barely seemed to notice that the more we vomited ourselves into emptiness, the more we needed to eat. It seemed a harmless way to keep our weight down. We had no idea that what we were playing with was anything but harmless. For some, this starve/binge/vomit cycle proves fatal. For several of us at my school, it was the beginning of a nightmarish addiction that would undermine our lives for decades to come—an addiction as dangerous as alcohol or drugs, and perhaps as difficult to overcome.

It had a name even then. But I wasn't to discover the word "bulimia" until I began writing my first *Workout Book* in 1981. I had thought for years that this bizarre practice was something only I and a few friends had stumbled upon. Today, of course, bulimia as well as anorexia has reached epidemic proportions. And they've both become subjects of national concern.

Bulimia is an illness, just as alcoholism is an illness. It may begin as a device to keep you from gaining weight and seem innocuous enough at first. Like alcoholism, however, it takes on a life of its own, consuming you until your life is out of control. The purging becomes an end in itself, more important than the food which is eaten but not always enjoyed. The bulimic finds herself more and more isolated. While her health suffers, so do her relationships. Intimacy becomes impossible.

The reasons for bulimia are many. A biochemical imbalance can leave a person physically vulnerable to bulimia. Certainly, there are psychological

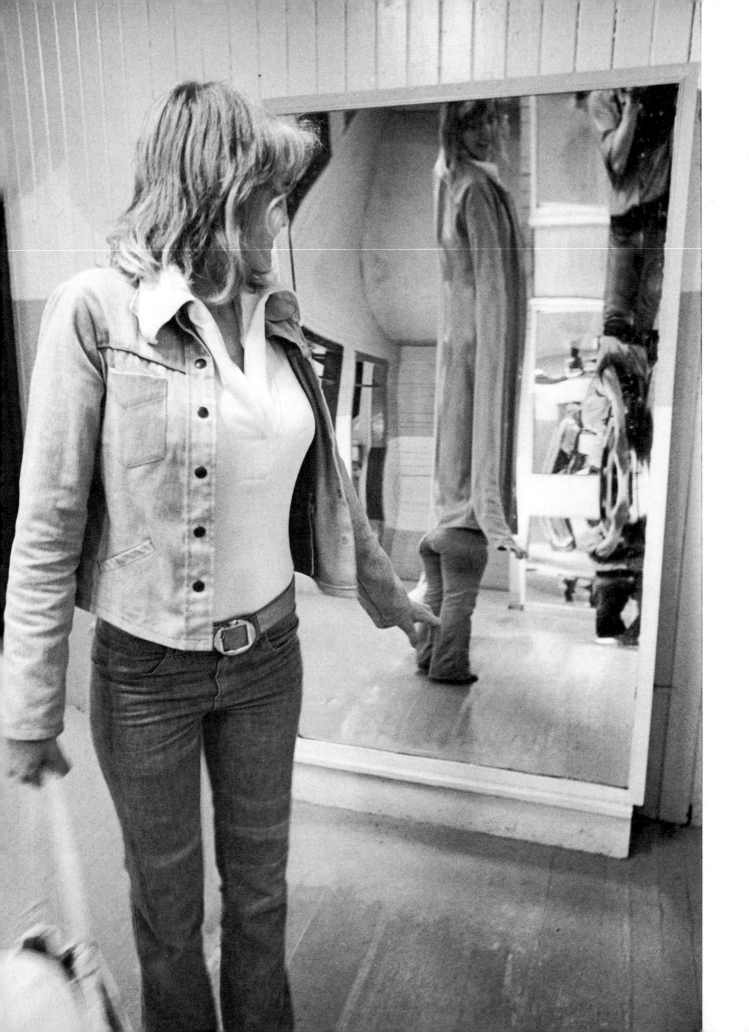

problems involved in this illness as well, problems beyond the social pressures to be thin. But just as an alcoholic must first stop drinking before she can begin to probe the underlying problems that led to her addiction, so too must the bulimic break the destructive cycle before the root causes can be addressed. The binging and vomiting have to stop first. In their place, a normal, structured eating pattern has to be introduced as part of any successful treatment.

It is usually advisable for anyone suffering from bulimia to seek professional help. Remember, this is a serious, complex disease. While most bulimics can recover, the recovery is not something best attempted alone. Remember too that, like alcoholism, bulimia is progressive. The longer it is allowed to continue, the worse the illness becomes and the harder it is to treat.

Usually, though not always, treatment is a difficult and protracted process. In her book *Bulimia: The Binge-Purge Compulsion*, psychotherapist Janice Cauwels describes how bulimics come to her wanting a quick "cure" when real recovery takes careful time. "A year of abstinence is probably a fair estimate of success," she states, "although I have one patient who re-

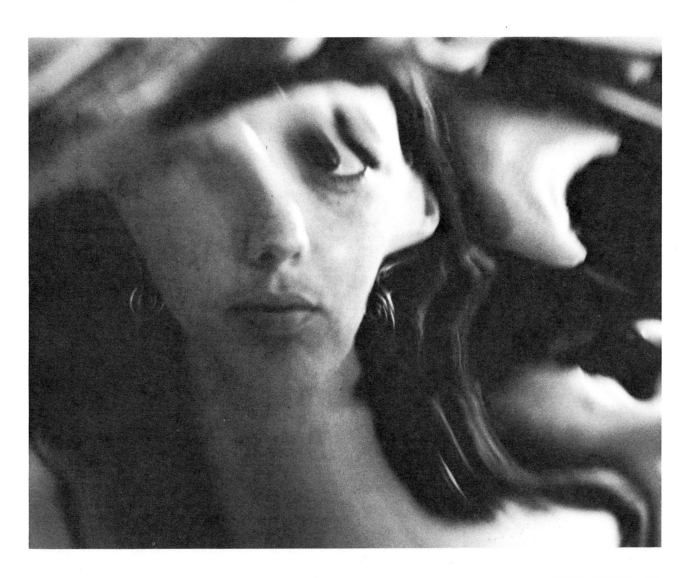

lapsed even after that long a period of abstinence. Bulimia is like cancer or tuberculosis in that it can be arrested and seem 'cured' after a specific period of remission, but the danger of relapse always remains."

Critical to recovery is the bulimic's motivation and her willingness to accept responsibility for stopping the destructive behavior. With treatment, a bulimic will learn to recognize and avoid the things that trigger a binge, to express her feelings and handle stress better, and to develop a stable eating structure she can rely on. The more distance the bulimic puts between herself and her binge-purge habit, the easier it becomes to eat in a healthy way until, in time, she can assume a less rigid, more spontaneous relationship with food and with her weight.

As I have already noted, the study of bulimia is still relatively new. No one can claim complete knowledge of its causes or its "cures." This much is clear, however: with proper treatment, most bulimics can recover totally or at least see substantial improvement.

No one form of treatment appears to be right for everyone. For some bulimics, individual therapy with a therapist who specializes in eating disorders will prove successful. For others, group therapy is most effective. Today, for most, a combination of individual *and* group therapy is advised. (If particularly acute, bulimia sometimes requires hospitalization in a special eating disorders unit.)

If you or a loved one need to find an eating specialist, whether for bulimia or for anorexia, try calling the largest hospital or medical school near your home. Many universities in various parts of the country have established eating disorders clinics to provide expert care while furthering research on this problem. In the reference section at the back of the book, I have listed these clinics as well as a number of eating disorders organizations you can contact for help. The American Anorexia Nervosa Association runs self-help groups around the country for those who cannot afford therapy or who want to supplement their private treatment. These groups are for anorexics and bulimics alike. The Anorexia Association also runs groups for parents and families, much as AA's Al-Anon program does for the parents and families of alcoholics. Overeaters Anonymous is another self-help organization that uses AA techniques to help people stop compulsive eating.

If you are bulimic, I advise you to tell the people close to you right away. This step—making it harder for you to get away with your covert behavior —can be your first step toward stopping. It may also provide you with the support you need in finding help. If you suspect bulimia in someone you care about, confront the person and encourage him or her to seek treatment. Remind whoever it is—your friend, your child, your partner, yourself—that bulimia is an illness. Bulimia doesn't make them, or you, a weak or bad person.*

* I would like to express my appreciation to Dr. Michael Strober, Director of the Teenage Eating Disorders Program at the U.C.L.A. Neuropsychiatric Institute, for his assistance on the issue of bulimia, and my admiration for the pioneering work being done by his program.

# FAT VERSUS WEIGHT:
# THE CRUCIAL DIFFERENCE

Quite apart from our overemphasis on thinness as an esthetic ideal, the very real problem of excess weight threatens one out of every three Americans. Sixty to seventy million adults and ten million teenagers are overweight. Aside from their emotional and psychological problems, people who have a great deal of extra body fat run greater risks of heart disease, high blood pressure, diabetes, and some forms of cancer.

The problem, however, is less one of being over*weight* than it is of being over*fat*. Many of us may actually not be overweight and yet have a higher percentage of body fat in relation to our lean body mass (muscle, bones and tissues of our organs) than is healthy.

Doctors say that normal percentages of fat are 12 to 15 percent for men, and 18 to 24 percent for women. Obesity, according to definition, exists when more than 20 percent of body weight is composed of fat in men and 25 percent or more in women. At these levels it becomes imperative for people to reduce their body fat and increase their lean body mass. The lower limit of fatness for most healthy women is about 12 percent of their total body weight.

There are several ways to determine your percentage of body fat. The simplest but least accurate, unless performed by a well-trained technician, is to take skin-fold measurements with a caliper, measuring fat under the skin at various sites such as the back of the arm, hip, shoulder blade, stomach, and leg. Caliper measurements can be off either way by 3 percent.

An accurate but rather impractical method of determining body fat is hydrostatic (underwater) weighing, in which your weight on land is compared to your weight taken under water.

Another quite accurate and easily administered technique, which we use at the Workout, sends a very mild ultrasound wave through the body at mid-thigh and waist, reading the thickness of body fat at those points. From this information, combined with your basic statistics, the computer determines the percentage and weight of your body fat, and the percentage and weight of your lean tissue, as well as a number of other health-related statistics. Unlike electrical impedance, another method used to measure body fat, ultrasound measures accurately, regardless of recent food eaten or water consumed.

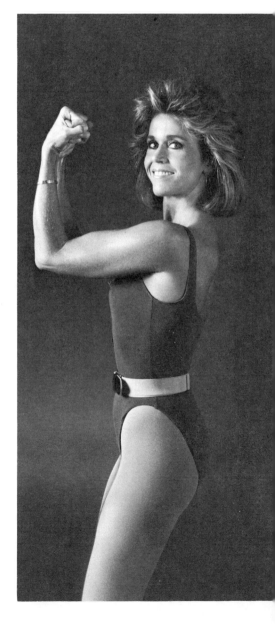

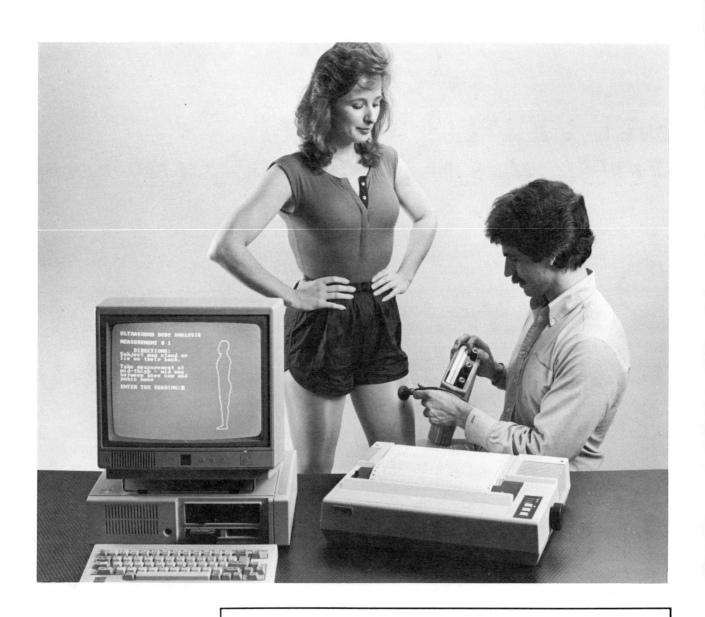

## MEASURING YOUR BODY FAT

Ultrasound: Price range is $5.00 to $20.00. Can be obtained at local fitness programs, Y.M.C.A.'s, sports medicine clinics, and health spas.

Skinfold Calipers: Price range is $5.00 to $35.00. Can be obtained at sports medicine clinics, health spas, local cardiac rehabilitation programs, and most hospitals that have wellness programs, sports medicine centers, or cardiac programs.

Hydrostatic Weighing: Price range is $15.00 to $50.00. Can be obtained at many university hospitals that offer wellness programs or preventive medicine, cardiac rehabilitation, or sports medicine programs. Hydrostatic weighing is most often accompanied by a treadmill or cycle ergometer test.

When we speak of wanting to "lose weight," what we should really be working for is to lose body fat while maintaining lean body mass, or muscle.

Most of the methods that we have tended to use in order to lose weight have, without our even realizing it, been counterproductive—sometimes chronically so. My purpose here is to explain why and to give you a basic understanding of what a rational, effective *fat*-loss program should look like.

## METABOLISM

To start off, it is necessary to have a basic understanding of our metabolism, the internal combustion that takes place in our body cells when already digested fats, proteins and carbohydrates (in the form of glucose) are "burned" to create energy—with the help of oxygen. The energy released is measured in calories.

About one third to one half of the energy we metabolize is energy that is used to keep the body functioning, the brain, heart, and other muscles and organs working while we are awake but resting. This energy is called our *basal metabolism,* and it is higher in men than in women.

During the day as we exercise or just go about our lives, we increase our output of energy over and above our basal metabolism through the use of our muscles. Muscles compose the largest part of the body and, together with the bones, make up our lean body mass. The muscles are an *active* tissue, burning, like furnaces, 90 percent of all the body's calories. Fat, on the other hand, is *inert.* Fat stored in the body doesn't burn calories, and they use up these calories even while we are resting. Fat *is* calories. Once you understand this, you will see that as the ratio of lean body mass to body fat increases, the number of calories used in metabolism increases.

This helps explain the phenomenon of middle-age spread. As we get older we tend to put on weight. While this is partly due to the fact that we tend to be less active as we age yet eat the same amount, it is also attributable to the fact that we lose, on the average, 3 to 5 percent of our muscle tissue each decade after 30. This results in a slowing of our basal metabolism—unless, of course, our habits change and we consciously work to increase our muscle mass and eat fewer (but more nutrient-rich) calories.

The body's ability to store fat is unlimited. On the other hand, we can store only a limited amount of carbohydrates and protein. When we surpass these limits by eating more than we need they are stored as fat. To give you a dramatic example: if you eat just 100 calories more than you use up every day, you can expect to gain more than 50 pounds in five years. This happens unnoticeably at first, with the stored fat penetrating the muscle itself and replacing the lean muscle tissue. Once the muscle is saturated, fat is next deposited subcutaneously—that is, in adipose tissue under the skin. In order to lose these deposits of subcutaneous fat one must use them up as a source of energy. To do this, the number of calories of food eaten must be less than the number of calories burned up as energy. The additional energy needed during the day will have to come from the stored fat.

Of course, all bodies don't function in exactly the same way. Some people utilize food energy less efficiently than others and have a greater tendency

*Taking a skin-fold measurement of subcutaneous fat with a caliper*

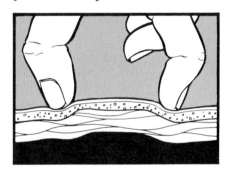

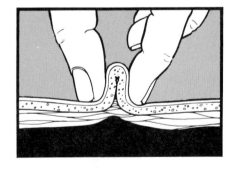

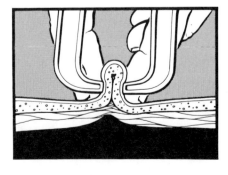

to store fat. There can also be a great variance in the basal metabolic rate from person to person. Furthermore, it is now believed that the temperature in the hypothalamus gland within the brain may actually control our appetite. This theory says the specific heat given off during digestion causes a stimulation in the part of the brain that tells us when we're full. This may explain why people's appetites increase in the cold and decrease in the heat. It may also explain why exercise, which heats up our bodies, has a short-term depressant effect on the appetite.

These are some of the reasons why one person tends to get fat while eating modestly, yet another, eating the same amount and equally active or inactive, will lose weight.

Generally speaking, however, it is absolutely possible to alter your metabolism by building and maintaining the active tissues of your muscles. This is most safely and effectively done when exercise that burns fat stores and increases muscle mass is combined with a weight-loss diet designed to use up excess fat with minimal loss of lean muscle tissue.

# UNDERSTANDING THE BASICS

Most people's knowledge of food doesn't extend beyond their sense of taste. They know what they like and that's about it. But food is more than a matter of taste: it's the stuff we're made of. It's the energy we run on. The food you eat affects every cell in your body, and, as I've discovered the hard way, it affects the way you feel each day. It never occurs to most of us that a poor diet can be responsible for fatigue, headaches, irritability, digestive problems, and similar troubles that have nothing to do with weight. But when you begin to think of food as essential fuel for a delicately balanced machine—your body—you'll appreciate that indiscriminate eating can cause a host of physical and even emotional problems. It is only smart to gain an understanding of what constitutes the body's best raw materials and best fuel. It is merely common sense to acquire some nutritional know-how. The pleasures of eating, I assure you, will remain. You may even find them enhanced.

Six major nutrients come to us in food: proteins, carbohydrates, fats, vitamins, minerals, and water.

Each is *essential* and each interacts with the others. Once these nutrients enter the digestive system, enzymes and other substances help to transform the proteins into amino acids, the carbohydrates into glucose, and the fats into fatty acids. In these new forms, the major nutrients are absorbed into the bloodstream.

From the bloodstream, the fats go directly into the cells—as do the fat-soluble vitamins. The other nutrients go to the liver first, where their chemical composition changes even further, preparing them to be put to work in cell metabolism. Metabolism is the process by which digested nutrients are converted into energy or into building materials for the body's tissues. At all of these stages, enzymes act as catalysts that either start or hasten chemical reactions inside the body. All along the way, vitamins and minerals must be present for the enzymes to do their job properly.

**PROTEIN.** Protein's role is to build, repair, and maintain the cells of virtually every body tissue. It also supplies energy when the body's carbohydrate and fat reserves have been exhausted. Such depletion is not desirable, however, since protein *cannot* be stored and we need it twenty-four hours a day for building, repairing, and maintaining the skin, bones, muscles, organs, and all the rest. Protein also stimulates production of enzymes, hormones, and even the antibodies that fight infections for us. If we have to dip into our protein allowance for energy, these vital processes will suffer. (This is why any weight-loss program should ensure sufficient protein intake.)

Proteins are made up of amino acids. There are twenty-three of them altogether, fourteen of which are manufactured by the body itself. The other nine must be obtained from food. Animal proteins like fish, poultry, eggs, milk, and cheese give us *complete* protein with all nine of the essential amino acids that the body does not manufacture. Plant foods like rice, beans, wheat germ, seeds, and nuts contain protein too, but not all nine essential amino acids. These foods are *incomplete* proteins by themselves. But when properly combined, they form complete proteins. Rice combined with beans, for instance, provides the full nine amino acids, as do whole-grain cereals combined with milk and whole-grain breads with cheese.

Most of us were brought up to believe that we need large amounts of protein and that the best way to get it is to eat a lot of meat. The health consequences of this kind of diet are becoming evident today. People regularly eat twice as much protein as they need, largely through overconsumption of beef. We're learning more about the drawbacks of this diet all the time. Too much meat is unquestionably unhealthful. And too much protein is as unhealthful as too little. We know now that we'll do our bodies the greatest good by getting *most* of our protein from plant rather than animal sources. (I'll discuss this in greater detail in the next chapter.)

How much protein is enough? For most of us, *35 to 55 grams a day* is ample. Your own protein requirements undoubtedly fall within this range. To calculate your needs exactly, here is an easy formula to use. The recommended dietary allowance or RDA for protein is .36 grams per pound of body weight. Multiply your specific body weight by .36. The result will tell you how many grams of protein you should eat every day. (A 120-pound woman requires 43 grams, for example, according to this formula.) To get a sense of the amount of protein in the foods you eat, you'll need to consult a food composition chart at first.* You'll find, for instance, that a 3-½ oz. breast of chicken contains 23 grams of protein and the same amount of cod has 18 grams. Fortunately, many packaged products list their protein content on the outside. My carton of milk, for instance, tells me that an 8-ounce glass of milk contains 10 grams of protein. My carton of cottage cheese lists a half-cup as having 14 grams.

**CARBOHYDRATES.** Carbohydrates are our chief source of energy. They are readily digested and converted into glucose, which is the form of sugar found in the bloodstream and often referred to as blood sugar. Glucose provides energy for the brain, the nervous system, and the muscles. It works like a fire's kindling, helping the body to burn the denser fuel of fat more efficiently. A limited amount of glucose is stored in the muscles and liver as

---

* Composition charts can be found in many nutrition and diet books. You can also request a copy of the "Nutritional Composition of Foods" by writing to the U.S. Government Printing Office at:

    Superintendent of Documents
    U.S. Government Printing Office
    Washington, D.C. 20402

the reserve fuel known as glycogen. But any excess of glucose is stored as fat.

Carbohydrates come in two forms: simple and complex. The simple carbohydrates are sugars and are rapidly broken down into glucose and absorbed by the blood. These give us an immediate energy jolt followed by an equally sudden energy drop. Much better for us are the complex carbohydrates. Made up of starches and fibers, these break down into glucose more slowly. This means they provide more sustained energy over a greater length of time than do the simple carbohydrates. Unless refined and depleted of nutrients through food processing, the complex carbohydrates are a treasure trove of vitamins and minerals, as well as of indigestible fibers that help to keep our digestive tracts clean and healthy, and that also help to slow our rate of glucose absorption.

**FAT.** Fat is the second most important energy source. As our most concentrated form of energy, it's the fuel you train your body to burn during long sessions of aerobic exercise that draw on your body's endurance. Fat also insulates you, lubricates the cells, protects the skin and other tissues from dryness, and assists the body in its absorption of the fat-soluble vitamins.

Fats exist in both saturated and unsaturated forms. Saturated fat is usually solid at room temperature and is derived principally from animals. (Think of butter and lard.) Unsaturated fat is usually liquid at room temperature and comes largely from the oils of vegetables, seeds, and nuts.

The solid saturated fats contain *cholesterol*. Cholesterol, which made the cover of *Time* magazine last year, is a waxy fatlike substance that's necessary for good health but that's strongly associated, in excess, with chronic artery disease and chronic heart disease. Unsaturated fats, on the other hand, have *no* cholesterol. They are preferable to saturated fats for this reason, as well as for being our *only* source of the one essential fatty acid, linoleic acid. *One tablespoon of vegetable oil a day provides our daily requirement for linoleic acid.*

It's important to know, however, that even the unsaturated fats are troublesome in excess. You should also know that some are less unsaturated than others. Coconut and palm oils, for instance, are nearly solid—even at room temperature. Commonly found as ingredients in processed foods, these are always best avoided.

**VITAMINS.** Vitamins are chemicals that assist the proteins, fats, and carbohydrates in fulfilling their different functions in the body. Vitamins themselves provide no energy or calories. Rather, as components of enzymes, they help to metabolize other nutrients into energy—the fats and carbohydrates. Likewise, they help to convert proteins into the building blocks of the cells. Vitamins participate in all the biochemical reactions inside us. They even assist in the formation of nervous system and brain chemicals, some of which are known to influence our moods.

There are two main types of vitamins: water-soluble and fat-soluble. Those soluble in water can't be stored in the body, and we must continually replenish them by eating foods that provide them. These are vitamin C and the B-complex vitamins. Fat-soluble vitamins *are* stored in the body. These are vitamins A, D, E, and K. (In excess, these can build to toxic levels, but this happens rarely.)

**MINERALS.** Minerals are as life-sustaining and vital to your overall mental and physical well-being as vitamins. We have minerals in all our body tissues and fluids—in our blood, bones, teeth, and skin, for example. The minerals work along with the vitamins to assist in food metabolism. They also participate in transmitting nerve messages, contracting and releasing the muscles, producing hormones, and regulating the body's fluid balance. Too much sodium, for instance, will cause us to retain water.

The *major* minerals present in relatively high amounts in the body are calcium, magnesium, potassium, phosphorus, sodium, chlorine, and sulfur. The *trace* minerals present in the most minute but equally essential quantities are iron, zinc, selenium, iodine, manganese, copper, chromium, fluoride, and several others.

While vitamins are quite fragile, minerals are far less so. The major and the trace minerals are rarely missing from our diet, with the serious exception of *calcium, iron,* and *zinc.* Women, for example, chronically get too little calcium. This deficiency can result in the brittle bones of osteoporosis in the later years of life. I'll talk more about this later.

**WATER.** Water is *the* primary nutrient—second only to oxygen as a prerequisite for life. The body can withstand the absence of food much longer than it can the absence of water!

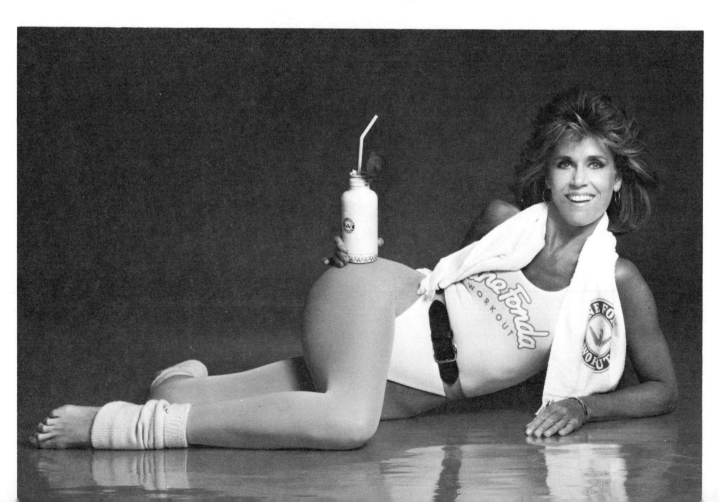

## THE RIGHT BALANCE

- *Complex Carbohydrates*
  These are the *main course* of a healthy, high-energy diet. Of the total calories you consume daily, 60–75 percent should be complex carbohydrates.

- *Proteins*
  Protein should represent 15–20 percent of your total daily calories. This is your diet's essential *condiment*.

- *Fats*
  These should constitute the *smallest portion* of a healthy diet—a little oil for flavor and for essential linoleic acid. Fats can provide as little as 10 percent of your daily calories. They should provide *no more* than 25 percent. Less is always best. (The 25 percent figure is deceptively high when compared to actual quantities of the other food groups. This is because fat has *twice* the calories of either carbohydrates or proteins.)

## THE RIGHT SOURCES

- *Complex Carbohydrates*
  Vegetables
  Fruits
  Legumes: fresh and dried beans, peas, and lentils
  Whole grains: rice, wheat, corn, oats, and barley (bread, pasta, and cereals made from whole grains)
  Seeds: in moderation
  Nuts: in moderation

- *Proteins*
  Fish: without the skin
  Poultry: without the skin
  Milk: low-fat and nonfat
  Yogurt: low-fat and nonfat
  Cheeses: low-fat cottage cheese, mozzarella, feta, ricotta, and farmer's cheese
  Eggs: in moderation
  Combinations of complementary proteins: legumes, whole grains, seeds, nuts, and some vegetables and dairy products
  Tofu (bean curd, a soybean product from the legume family)

- *Fats*
  Vegetable oils: corn, safflower, sunflower, and soybean oils (peanut, olive, and sesame oils, sparingly)

Water is present in every cell and constitutes *two-thirds* of your body weight. You need it for virtually every body function. It flushes wastes away, cools us through sweat, keeps the skin and mucous membranes moist, and much more. Fresh fruits and vegetables are excellent sources. Nearly every fruit, for example, is 90 percent pure water—dark green, leafy vegetables too. In addition to eating plenty of these foods, we need to drink lots of water too—a good six to eight glasses a day.

You now have, in brief form, a basic blueprint of the six major nutrients needed by the body. These help determine how well your complex biochemistry functions. They influence how efficiently your trillions of cells rejuvenate themselves. They can make all the difference in whether you limp through your days with debilitating highs and lows or whether you ride confidently on a steady, sustained stream of energy.

# THE RIGHT STUFF

Today, 62 percent of the calories we consume come from sugar, animal fat, and alcohol. Each of these is bereft of nutrients, which means that well over *half* the food we're eating has *no* nutritive value whatsoever! This is the Standard American Diet—the low-nutrient, low-fiber, high-fat, high-sugar, and high-calorie SAD diet. As a society, we couldn't be digging our graves with our forks any faster.

There has to be a changing of the dietary guard—and, fortunately, it appears to have begun. The harmful highs have to become healthful lows—low fat, low sugar, low calorie. The old lows have to become new highs—high nutrient, high fiber. These are all part of what I call The Right Stuff—the principles that form the foundation of our changing nutritional menu. These are the best guidelines you can have for creating a healthy diet for yourself and for your family.

---

**THE RIGHT STUFF**

1. Cut down on meat.
2. Substitute low-fat for high-fat foods.
3. Cut down on sugar.
4. Avoid salt and salty foods.
5. Eat fewer processed foods.
6. Emphasize the complex carbohydrates.
7. Take a multivitamin and mineral supplement.
8. Drink plenty of water.
9. Drink little alcohol and caffeine.
10. Seek lots of variety in food.
11. Go for balance and moderation.

---

## 1. Cut down on meat.

Meat is not without its virtues. It's a solid source of protein. And it's full of iron. However, the benefits of eating meat and to a lesser extent other animal proteins unquestionably fail to outweigh the problems:

• Most meat is very high in fat—especially saturated fat—and cholesterol.
• Virtually all beef and poultry today comes from animals raised in high-tech feedlots. Their meat contains synthetic hormones, pesticide residues, antibiotics, and other undesirable chemicals.

Deer and antelope may be the only animals still home on the range these days. The cattle that once roamed the range are now crammed flank to flank under the glare of round-the-clock artificial lights. In the days when cattle

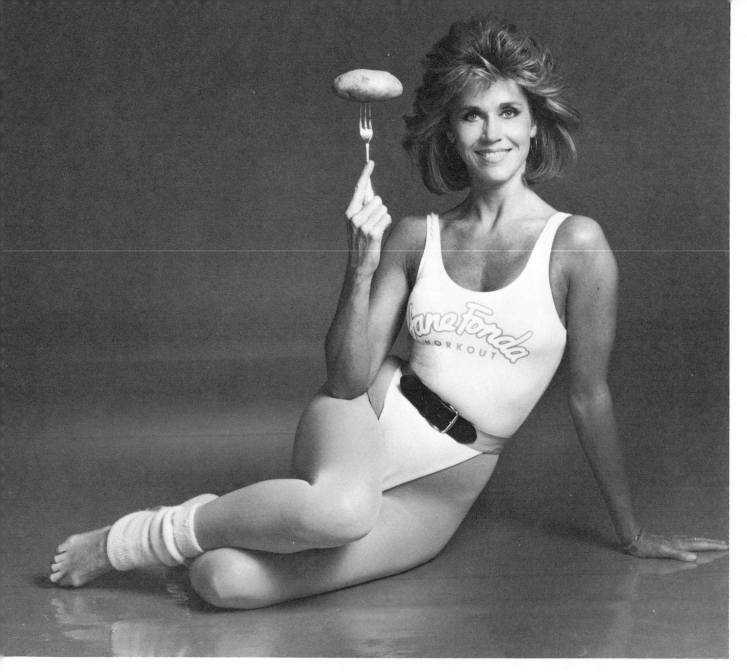

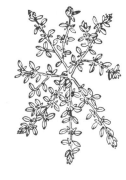

grazed, they weren't considered mature enough for slaughter until they were three or four years old. Today, in the feedlots, cattle are fattened quickly and cheaply and slaughtered in half that time. The fat of livestock that roamed freely and matured naturally was largely unsaturated. The fat of feedlot cattle is almost entirely saturated.

This kind of meat production results in high profits, but it also subjects the animals to stress and to an increased risk of disease. To minimize these problems, antibiotics and tranquilizers are routinely administered. It is estimated that close to 90 percent of the cows and chickens raised for market in this country have received antibiotics and other drugs since birth. Synthetic hormones and other chemicals are also added to livestock feed in order to stimulate growth and weight gain. The residues are often found in animal tissues. They're *not* eliminated through cooking. All of this is of concern to health authorities. Among other things, they fear that our routine exposure to antibiotics in meat will render these drugs ineffective if the time comes when we need them to fight off certain human illnesses. Harmful microbes are known to build a tolerance to antibiotics as a result of such prolonged exposure.

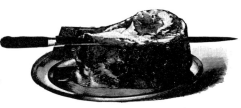

What is to be done?

First and foremost, try to eat less meat, especially red meat.

Second, eat less processed, cured, smoked, and charred meats—and also less liver. All of these are chemical quagmires.

Third, if you do eat meat, seek out beef and poultry from animals that have been raised naturally. Whenever possible, for example, I buy what are called free-range chickens. Most commercially sold chickens have been raised indoors in such a confined space that they can hardly move. They have never been out in the sunshine or seen a rooster. They've been fed on chemical mush. And their eggs are infertile. Free-range chickens, on the other hand, are raised outdoors. They feed on grains, seeds, insects, and worms. They're given no synthetic foods or chemicals. Raised with roosters, these chickens produce fertile eggs, which have a higher vitamin content. And their meat contains less saturated fat and provides more nutritional value than that of poultry raised in commercial brooders.

If you can't find a butcher, health-food store, or other source for such naturally raised chickens or for naturally raised cattle, try at least to buy your meat *fresh*. Insist on beef being cut in your presence and be sure the excess fat is trimmed.

Fourth, remember that non-meat sources of protein abound—low-fat dairy products, fish, and combinations of plant proteins that complement each other. If your basic diet consists of whole non-junk foods, getting enough protein without meat is far easier than has commonly been believed.

## 2. Substitute Low-fat for High-fat Foods.

As stated in the previous chapter, fats should be the smallest portion of a healthy diet. Yet, the diet of the average American is over 40 percent fat! Of the fatty foods most commonly eaten, meat heads the list. It's followed by whole milk, ice cream, whole-milk cheeses, and butter—in that order. As you can see, the favored fats are the saturated ones, the fats strongly associated with high levels of cholesterol. Such a high-fat, high-cholesterol diet is linked to *all* the major chronic diseases—especially atherosclerosis, heart disease, cancer, and colon cancer. Because fats are so loaded with calories, empty calories at that, high-fat diets also mean problems with weight.

I can't recommend strongly enough that you eat less fat, and especially less saturated fat. Cutting down on red meat is a giant step in this direction.

Here are a few other ways to trim fat from your diet:

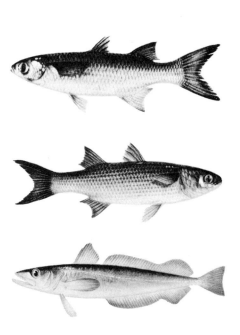

- If you do eat meat, always choose the leanest cuts.
- Use meat more as a condiment than as a main course.
- Use nonfat and low-fat dairy products—milk, yogurt, and cheese.
- Limit your eggs to two a week (one egg alone has so much cholesterol in its yolk that it brings you nearly to the recommended daily maximum of 300 mg).

- In cooking:
  - Trim all fat from meat first.
  - Take the skin off poultry and fish (and select their least fatty forms).
  - Broil, poach, or steam—don't fry.
  - Use a nonstick skillet that makes oil less necessary.
  - Substitute vegetable oils for saturated fats like lard and butter.
- Use vegetable oils in moderation. (*Always* refrigerate your oils in order to protect them from the process of oxidation, which causes rancidity. Rancid oils promote internal chemical damage. The fresher the oil, the healthier).
- Familiarize yourself with cholesterol's "10 Most Unwanted List" (opposite).

---

## GETTING COMPLETE PROTEIN WITHOUT MEAT

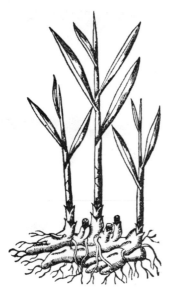

*The Basic Combinations*

1. Whole grains (rice, wheat, corn, oats, barley, and their products)
   +
   Legumes (fresh or dried beans, peas, and lentils)

2. Whole grains
   +
   Dairy products* (milk, yogurt, and cheese)

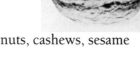

3. Nuts and seeds (black walnuts, peanuts, pine nuts, cashews, sesame seeds, and sunflower and pumpkin seeds)
   +
   Legumes

* Dairy products maximize the protein in *all* plant foods.

---

### 3. Cut down on sugar.

Sugar is like fat's twin—tied to excess weight and to the same laundry list of chronic diseases. It's also our *number one food additive!* With sugar laced into so many products on grocery shelves, no wonder Americans are so hooked on sweets. Eating lots of sweets wreaks havoc on the body and keeps us craving more.

Sugar is a simple carbohydrate. Burning simple carbohydrates for fuel is like burning newspaper for heat. Both ignite with a bright flame, but the flame quickly dies. And then more paper—more sugar—has to be added to keep the fire going. It's a vicious cycle as far as sugar is concerned. Too much sugar means your blood sugar levels will be riding a roller coaster that soars too high and plunges too low.

Here's what happens inside when we eat lots of sugar. A rush of glucose or blood sugar stimulates the pancreas to secrete high levels of the hormone insulin. The surge of insulin causes the rapid cell absorption of glucose from

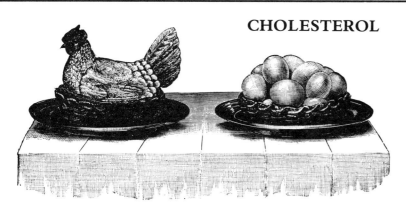

# CHOLESTEROL

## THE 10 MOST UNWANTED LIST

| | | Cholesterol/mg |
|---|---|---:|
| 1. | Chicken liver, 8 oz. | 1692 |
| 2. | Beef liver, 8 oz. | 418 |
| 3. | Egg, one | 274 |
| 4. | Veal, 8 oz. | 225 |
| 5. | Lamb, 8 oz. | 222 |
| 6. | Beef, all cuts, 8 oz. | 197–213 |
| 7. | Pork, all cuts, 8 oz. | 116–202 |
| 8. | Chicken, no skin, 8 oz. | 136 |
| 9. | Butter, 1 tablespoon | 31 |
| 10. | Cheeses,* 1 oz. | 14–32 |

Remember:
- The maximum recommended daily consumption of cholesterol is 300 mg.
- Vegetables, fruits, grains, and all other plant foods contain *no* cholesterol.

*The cheeses lowest in cholesterol are low-fat cottage cheese, ricotta, mozzarella, and provolone.

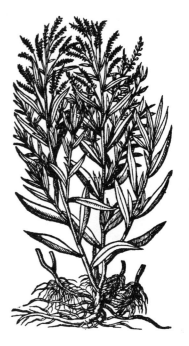

the blood. As a result, our blood sugar level drops quickly. Meanwhile, the insulin lingers in the blood, keeping the blood sugar down—and keeping us down along with it. We feel tired and sometimes depressed. So we're compelled to reach for the quick energy of more sugar. And so it goes. There's a little-known side effect too. The more insulin we secrete, the faster fat is also absorbed by the cells. By eating too much sugar, in other words, we're actually encouraging the body to store fat!

I recommend that you take sugar and sugary foods off your kitchen shelves. This goes for the brown and raw sugars, as well as for the white stuff. They're all simple sugars. They're all empty calories. If you must use a sweetener, substitute blackstrap molasses, honey, or maple syrup—but use these sparingly. They have some nutritive value, but they're simple sugars too. I suggest forgetting *artificial* sweeteners altogether—or at least using them in moderation. None has a clean bill of health, including the new NutraSweet. Besides, they keep our desire for sweet flavors high. Try training your sweet tooth to be satisfied with fruit or whole grains instead of sugar. I know it's a habit hard to break, but it can be done.

# THE CRUMBLING PILLARS OF SALT

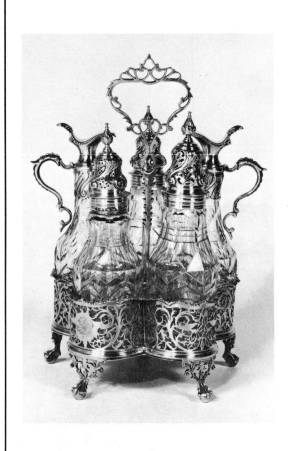

**Beware!**

Breakfast cereals, cold
   (with the exception of Puffed Wheat, Puffed Rice, Shredded Wheat, and some cereals found in natural food stores)
Baking soda and baking powder
Baking mixes
Gravy mixes
Canned vegetables
Canned soups
Canned tomatoes, tomato sauce, and ketchup
Chicken and beef bouillon cubes and powders
Frozen dinners
Fast foods (a Big Mac has 1,064 mg of sodium!)
Bacon, sausage, hot dogs, corned beef, and other cured meats
Pickles and pickled foods
Potato chips, pretzels, crackers, and other salty snack foods

Remember:
- The recommended *maximum* intake of sodium is 1200–3000 mg a day.
   (The body's actual requirement is only 220 mg a day.)
- 1 teaspoon of salt = 2,196 mg of sodium
   (1 teaspoon of soy sauce = 439 mg of sodium)
- Read package labels.
- Look for products labeled "no salt" and "low sodium."
- Ask restaurant chefs to "hold the salt—and the MSG."

## 4. Avoid salt and salty foods.

After sugar, salt is our number two food additive. Americans eat 20 to 30 times the salt the body actually needs! The health consequence is high blood pressure for one in six of us. High blood pressure often produces no symptoms at all until it has escalated into the crisis of a stroke, heart attack, or kidney failure. Another consequence of too much salt, less serious than high blood pressure but possibly more common, is water retention. This can result in a puffy appearance, a bloated feeling, a weight gain (a gain of water), and sometimes even depression.

I used to love salt and added it to everything. Then I went cold turkey during my first pregnancy. It was hard until I began discovering the subtle flavors in food that salt had been covering up. I've essentially lost my salt desire now. In fact, I find salt shocking to the taste buds. I no longer add salt to the food on my plate. Nor do I use salt when I cook. I recommend that you cut down on salt in the same ways. Don't worry that you won't be getting enough. There's plenty of sodium in the natural foods we eat. We're far more in danger of getting too much than too little.

Taking the salt shaker off the table and off the stove is a good first step. Eating fewer salty foods is another. I've listed the most common of these in the box that follows. Unfortunately, most cheeses are high in salt—especially the hard cheeses. So go easy on these. Among those lowest in salt are ricotta, mozzarella, Swiss, and Gruyere (some mozzarella is made with no salt at all). Your best bet in choosing any food that tends to be salty is to look for the label "salt-free" or "low-sodium." Fortunately, we'll be seeing a lot more of these words in our supermarkets.

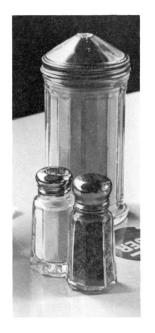

You'll probably find that eliminating salt means wanting to know more about the art of seasoning. It's a skill I'm still learning. We all have to feel and taste our way along as we settle on a few seasoning staples. I always have a pepper mill handy for grinding fresh black pepper, for instance, and cayenne pepper is also a staple (always add cayenne last in cooking because heat lessens its potency). Then, of course, there's garlic (fresh always), ginger, curry powder, chili powder, paprika, and many other fresh herbs and dried spices to experiment with. My family and I favor a powdered herbal and vegetable blend called "Veg-it," which we use as a salt substitute. In moderation, soy sauce is a good alternative from time to time, especially for stir-fried vegetables and rice. Soy sauce is actually a form of salt, but it contains much less sodium than table salt. Its flavor is stronger too, so you tend not to use as much. (One-quarter teaspoon of soy sauce gives the same seasoning power as one full teaspoon of table salt.) Natural soy sauces without preservatives are best (be sure to keep them refrigerated). Some are even marked "mild" or "low-sodium," though these are harder to find in the stores.

## 5. Eat fewer processed foods.

Cutting down the processed foods in your life will take you a long way toward subtracting the fat-sugar-salt trio from your diet—as well as a large measure of troublesome chemicals. (If you cut down on red meat too, you're almost home nutritionally.) If you give yourself a little time, you will develop a real preference for foods as close to their natural living state as possible. How much more pleasurable a cold, juicy, fresh peach than a soggy, sugary, syrupy canned one!

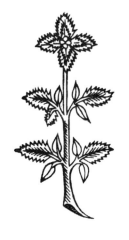

It's important to understand that some processed foods are less harmful than others. So please make it your habit to *read the labels first* when you do buy them. The ingredients are right there on the package. All labels list their ingredients in the descending order of amounts. In other words, the closer an item is to the top of the list, the greater the amount of that ingredient. The closer to the bottom, the smaller the amount.

Now, here are the major things to look for.

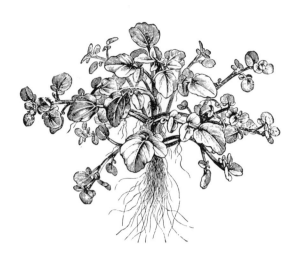

- *Additive number one—sugar*. Large quantities of sugar are hidden as sucrose, dextrose, fructose, corn syrup, beet sugar, and invert sugar in processed foods. You should know that commercially prepared breakfast cereals are notoriously high in sugar (even granola). Sugar is also high in most canned fruits, some canned vegetables, yogurts with fruit, salad dressings, breads, tomato sauces, ketchup, and many types of pickles, relishes, and condiments. When checking a label for sugar, don't forget to look for artificial sweeteners like saccharin and aspartame (or Nutra-Sweet). Remember, their health effects are uncertain.
- *Additive number two—salt*. Expect to see a lot of this. You'll know that a product contains salt any time you see the word "sodium." Monosodium glutamate or MSG is a common ingredient in processed foods, for instance. Because salt is a preservative, one of our oldest, it's present in cold cuts, bacon, hams, and other meats as sodium nitrites and sodium nitrates. (These present a danger besides their salt hazard: the body converts the nitrites and nitrates into nitrosamines, which are potential cancer-causing chemicals.)
- *Fat*. You can take it for granted that most snack and processed foods are loaded with dangerous fat. Watch out for coconut and palm oils, two vegetable oils that are almost totally saturated and should be avoided. Not all fats are bad, however. Olive oil, which is a monounsaturated fat, now appears to actually protect against heart disease by reducing the dangerous low-density lipoproteins that help cholesterol adhere to the walls of your blood vessels.

    Fish contains a special oil, called omega-3 fatty acid, that appears to help prevent blood clotting and to lower cholesterol levels. It is for this reason that many doctors are now recommending we eat some fish or fish oil capsules (cod liver or salmon oil) every day.
- *A range of questionable chemicals*. The following additives should be avoided:
    —the artificial colorings Citrus Red No. 2, Red No. 3, and Yellow No. 5
    —the artificial flavoring quinine (more testing needs to be done before this gets the green light)
    —the preservatives sodium nitrite, sodium nitrate, sulfur dioxide, and sodium bisulfite

—BHA or butylated hydroxyanisole
—BHT or butylated hydroxytoluene
—BVO or brominated vegetable oil
   (There's always the possibility of pesticide residues too, but of course that goes for fresh fruits and vegetables as well as processed foods.)

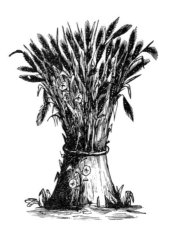

There's been conclusive evidence that many of these chemicals in food are risk factors for cancer—acting alone or in combination. The food industry argues in response that the doses administered to test animals are far larger than people would ever ingest. The assumption is that small doses of cancer-related substances pose no risk. Cancer experts disagree.

The development of cancer is complex, to say the least. In the vast majority of cases, there is no one cause. Rather, there's a constellation of interacting risk factors. Most toxic chemicals enter the body as *procarcinogens;* that is, they have to be activated in order to cause any damage. Other chemicals, neither procarcinogenic nor carcinogenic, enter the body as *promoters;* that is, they multiply the effects of already-existing toxins in the body. What is thought to ignite the fire of cancer is the interplay between such factors, the cumulative exposure to toxins, and the presence over prolonged periods of time of certain carcinogenic conditions like high-fat low-fiber diets, like smoking, like many summers of sunbathing.

When it comes to cancer, we'd be fools not to do all we can to control the *avoidable* risk factors in our lives—even if some of these are small risks in themselves, as the food industry claims is the case with food additives. There are enough carcinogens in the environment that we *can't* avoid. Take smog, for instance, or the growing problem of hazardous wastes and contaminated water. Why should we increase our risk of cancer one iota by knowingly ingesting even the tiniest amount of a questionable chemical?

## 6. Emphasize the complex carbohydrates.

These are foods that have sustained whole cultures for centuries. The hardiest, leanest athletes emphasize them, as do the peoples of the world known for their long lives. The complex carbohydrates should be central to your own nutritional life too: vegetables and legumes, fruits, whole-grain rice, pasta, cereals, and breads can easily supplant the old red meats, butter, hot dogs, pies, and cakes.

Complex carbohydrates are your energy base. They're loaded with vitamins and minerals. They're gentle on the body because they're digested more easily than animal foods. And they're your *only source of fiber.* Fiber is the residue from plant foods that the body can't digest or absorb. It's vital in toning the intestines for healthy, regular elimination, which protects you against constipation, hemorrhoids, and the more serious hazard of colon and rectal cancer. In addition, fiber slows down the digestion of carbohydrates, enabling their glucose to enter the system in a leisurely way. That's how these foods provide us with a steady supply of energy. In addition to slowing down our absorption of glucose, fiber also appears to decrease our absorption of fats. Calories as well as toxins are moved more speedily through the system.

When your diet is high in complex carbohydrates, as mine is, you'll know you're getting a goodly amount of fiber. Whole-wheat bread, for example, provides eight times the amount of fiber found in refined white bread.

## 7. Take a multivitamin and mineral supplement daily.

Taking supplements is one of the most controversial issues in nutrition today. Fortunately, research into this question is ongoing. Like many others, I've long advocated daily nutritional supplements as an insurance policy for obtaining *at least 100 percent of the RDAs*. Ideally, having a well-balanced diet is all most of us would ever need to ensure our getting the full range of vitamins and minerals. In fact, the food you eat is always the place to start. Food, your natural vitamin pill, should come first. No supplement can make up for poor or inadequate food choices.

Rarely, however, do the daily eating habits of most Americans fit the ideal pattern—even for those with the best intentions. In addition, it's hard to know how nutrient-rich even the freshest of foods are these days. If you recognize yourself in any of the following descriptions, you're likely to be running short on micronutrients and need to supplement your diet:

- You're single, tend not to cook for yourself, and have little variety in your day-to-day diet.
- Single or not, you're on the go most of the time, tend to eat erratically, and frequently settle for the convenience of fast foods.
- You're a casual vegetarian and tend to put little time into the planning and preparation of meals, getting most of your protein from eggs and cheese, getting little of your protein from other sources like beans, brown rice, or fish.
- You're always on a diet.
- You drink and/or smoke heavily.
- You exercise strenuously.

Whether you should take supplements beyond the multivitamins I'm recommending should be a careful decision—preferably one made with a nutritionally informed doctor who knows your health history. There is one nutrient in particular, however, which most women will find they need to supplement separately: the mineral *calcium*. Diets low in calcium are commonplace, I've learned. The average woman consumes far less than the recommended daily allowance. In fact, the average calcium deficiency is associated with significant bone loss and is believed to be one of the major causes of bones thinning to the breaking point—the disease known as osteoporosis, the most common and greatest health threat to women in their later years.

For both the prevention and treatment of osteoporosis, nutritionists and physicians alike now recommend that women consume *1,000 mg of calcium a day*—1,500 mg after natural menopause and after surgical menopause (the removal of the ovaries). (Exercise is also strongly recommended, incidentally.) Please check your own diet. If you determine that you are not getting the full recommended amount of calcium, increase your intake of calcium-rich foods. If you're still falling short, you'll need to begin the practice of taking a special calcium supplement. There are a variety of forms, so read the labels carefully when you go to purchase yours. Calcium carbonate is often recommended because it's the most concentrated form (you can take fewer tablets). Avoid bone meal and dolomite products because they contain potentially toxic levels of lead.

To get the most out of your calcium supplement, here are a few tips. (1) Divide your daily intake into several doses, saving the last for bedtime because we tend to lose more calcium during sleep (an added nighttime benefit: calcium is a mild natural tranquilizer). (2) Take your supplement in between meals, preferably, or with a little yogurt or milk. Try not to take calcium at the same time as fiber, such as bran, because fiber can decrease the amount of calcium that is absorbed through the intestine. (3) Your intake of magnesium should be half that of your calcium. So look for a supplement that contains calcium combined with magnesium, already properly balanced. (4) Vitamin D is essential for the absorption of calcium. If you're confined for some reason, and get absolutely no sunshine, you may want to use the calcium supplements on the market that come already combined with vitamin D. (If you have a history of kidney stones, be sure to consult your physician first.)

## 8. Drink plenty of water.

I've already sung the praises of water in previous pages. I try to drink six to eight glasses of water every day. It has restored my sense of well-being many, many times and helps me keep my weight down too. By the way, if you drink bottled sparkling water, you need to pay attention to its salt content. Be sure to choose the seltzers and waters marked no-salt.

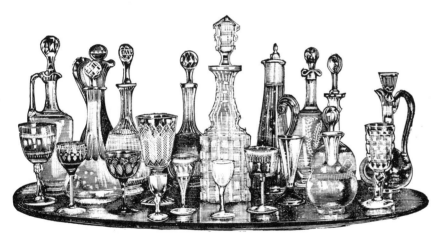

## 9. Drink little alcohol and caffeine.

Let's take the lesser of these two drugs first: caffeine. Caffeine is found in coffee, tea, many cola drinks, chocolate, and some aspirin-type painkillers. Caffeine is an unhealthful diuretic that depletes us of vitamin C, calcium, and many of the B vitamins, especially thiamine ($B_1$) and pantothenic acid ($B_5$). Caffeine gets our adrenaline pumping, as well as our insulin, which then plays havoc with the levels of sugar and fat in the blood. It produces an increased appetite, a craving for sweets, insomnia, nervousness, exhaustion, and also an exacerbation of fibrocystic breast conditions in women.

I've managed to stop drinking coffee, but it hasn't been easy. The smell of espresso in the morning was always like a good friend. But somehow the more coffee I drank, the more I felt I needed to renew my energy. Now that I'm clear of it, my energy is my own and my moods are more stable.

Now, for alcohol. Taken *in excess,* alcohol's ill effects are a lot like caffeine's—only the list is longer, more life-damaging, and potentially life-threatening.

Depression. Insomnia. A loss of nutrients—vitamin A, vitamin C, the B vitamins, as well as calcium and other minerals. Excessive blood fats. Highs *and* lows of blood sugar. And an accelerated aging process. Over time, alcohol taxes every major system of the body. It reaches every organ, and the liver and the brain are especially vulnerable. It's a well-known risk factor for heart disease, cancer, diabetes, and cirrhosis. And—it's addictive.

To any of you who may be unable to control your drinking, I strongly recommend that you contact Alcoholics Anonymous. Alcoholism is a disease. It worsens over time. And recovery is *highly unlikely* if you try to accomplish it alone. (There are local AA chapters everywhere across the country.)

For those of you with no addictive relationship to alcohol, alcohol can be okay—*in moderation.* This means a glass of wine, a beer, or a shot of hard liquor. In these moderate amounts, alcohol appears to be a mild tonic for the heart. Alcohol relaxes the blood vessels and is believed to raise the level of "healthy" fats in the blood known as HDLs, or high-density lipoproteins. This is especially the case for people who regularly exercise.

Don't forget, though. Alcohol is a drug. And even moderate amounts add 100 to 200 calories to your day's total. Like sugar and fat, these are nutritionally empty calories too.

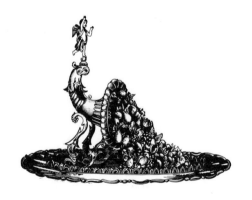

## 10. Seek lots of variety in foods.

Taking in an array of foods of different kinds and different colors is absolutely essential. Variety is the way to cover all your nutritional bases. Without it, you risk missing the full range of vitamins and minerals you need.

For people with busy lives (I suppose that's all of us), it's always easier to rely on our tried-and-true menus and the same old weekly shopping list. Staples may be good dietary anchors. But it's also important to keep our menu repertoires and eating patterns fresh. One way to do this is to spend a few extra minutes every week looking for a new menu to try and thinking about what vegetables, beans, or whole grains you haven't had in a while.

## 11. Go for balance and moderation.

Always.

# THE NEVER-FEEL-DEPRIVED DIET

The weight-loss diet I am recommending is not an off-again, on-again fad diet. In fact, I hope that you'll think of it not as the kind of restrictive diet you may be used to but rather as a new approach to eating and nutrition. My goal has been to make this diet as easy to live with as it is effective. That's why I call it the "Never-Feel-Deprived Diet." It won't leave you hungry and dissatisfied. This is because you'll be cutting calories gradually. And the foods you'll be encouraged to eat are largely complex carbohydrates.

Complex carbohydrates play the central role in my weight-loss diet. As you've learned, in addition to their wealth of nutrients these carbohydrates release glucose slowly into the bloodstream, which can minimize your hunger cravings and stabilize your energy and mood swings. What's more, the abundant fiber in complex carbohydrates will help you to feel full. Fiber is critical to losing weight. It is non-digestible bulk that satisfies hunger without adding calories to the diet. In fact, fiber helps to move calories more speedily through the body.

Recently, a study was done in which 35 college seniors were asked to eat only whole-grain foods and absolutely no white flour products for three months. By replacing the higher-calorie, low-fiber snack foods they had been accustomed to with lower-calorie, high-fiber foods, they lost an average of 17½ pounds each by the end of the three months! These students reported that the whole-grain foods began to appeal more to their taste as the study progressed.

While the Workout diet is weighted toward the fresh vegetables and starches of complex carbohydrates, it also provides all the protein you need in order to maintain your lean muscle tissue. And it does so without including dangerous fats and cholesterol.

I didn't invent this approach to dieting. More and more, experts in the field of nutrition and weight loss are advocating such low-fat, low-cholesterol, low-calorie, high-carbohydrate programs. But I do know from personal experience that they work.

Uncomplicated, easy to prepare, and inexpensive, this diet gives you the basics of a permanent way of eating—a diet for life. Once you achieve your proper weight, you can simply increase the size of the portions or add more starches and higher-calorie carbohydrates like fruits and nuts.

Starches, the complex carbohydrates such as rice, pasta, bread, and potatoes, have always been regarded as the stuff to stay away from when trying to lose weight. Yet, the *lack* of these nutrient-rich foods is what makes most

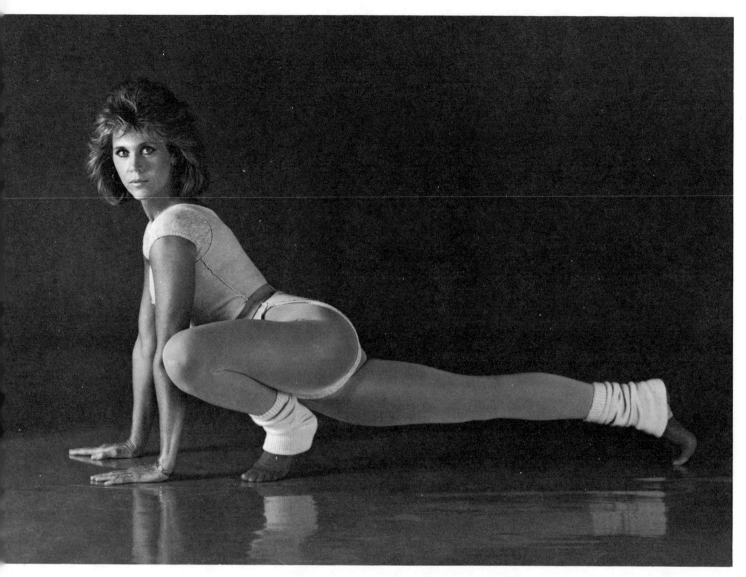

diets so unsatisfying and hard to stick to. Without them, we feel irritable and deprived most of the time. With them, we feel a sense of satiety as well as restfulness. (In part, this is due to the calming effect of the brain chemical serotonin, which is released when we eat carbohydrates.)

The truth is that starches are *not* fattening. In fact, they're *less* fattening than meat, which previously was always thought preferable for dieting. Just compare:

| | |
|---|---|
| 5 oz. steak | 5 oz. baked potato |
| *550* calories | *100* calories |
| | 5 oz. rice |
| | *153* calories |
| | 5 oz. pasta |
| | *210* calories |
| | 2 slices whole-wheat bread |
| | *120* calories |

## HOW TO DO IT

I have divided the foods you will be eating into their respective categories: Complex Carbohydrates, Proteins, Dairy, and Fats.

I've provided lists of each of these four food categories for you. These aren't intended to be inclusive but they do cover a wide variety of most of the lower-calorie, low-fat, high-nutrient foods you should eat. These are the foods you should emphasize.

Gradually cut back the number of calories you consume until you are taking in between 1,000 and 1,200 a day. But don't cut back by more than 500 calories a day from your ideal normal diet. If you cut too many calories too quickly it will be harder to stick to the diet.

Divide these calories *daily* among the four groups:

1. *Complex Carbohydrates*
   Two choices of dark green vegetables
   One choice another vegetable
   One or two choices of fruit (If only one, choose a citrus)
   Two choices from the cereal, bread, and grain category
2. *Proteins*
   One choice of fish or poultry; or beans combined with whole grains, nuts, or seeds (see page 34)
   One choice of meat *once or twice a week only*
3. *Dairy (a category of protein)*
   Two choices
4. *Fats*
   One choice

Make sure you include *all* of these choices every day. While there's an emphasis on vegetables, the diet must represent a *balance* between carbohydrates, proteins, and fats. Besides being good nutritional common sense, this way of eating will ensure that the protein in your muscles is protected as you lose weight.

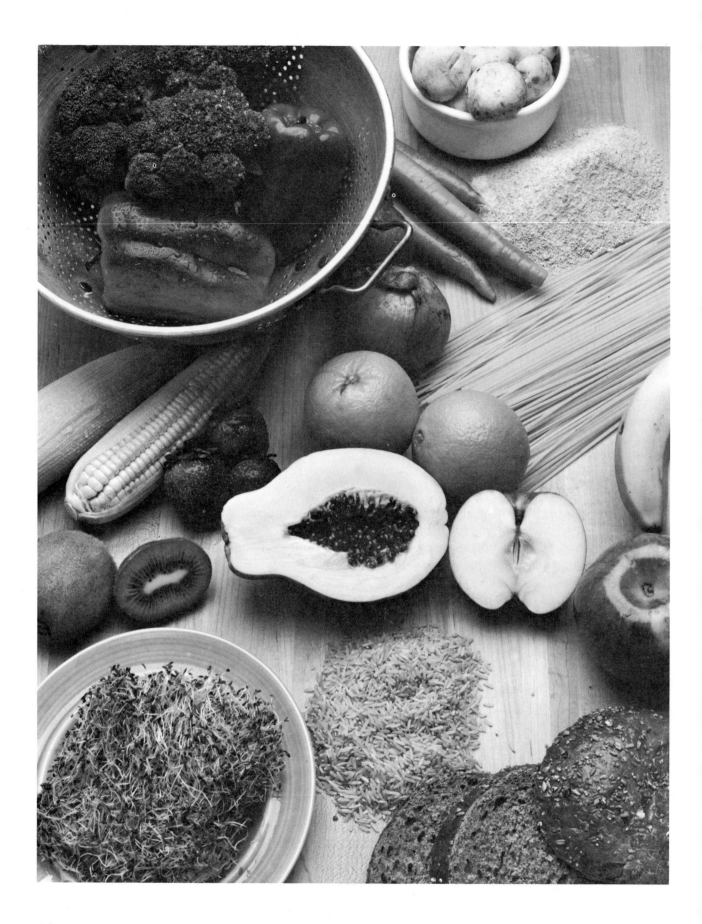

# FREE-CHOICE LIST

## Complex Carbohydrates

### Vegetables—Dark Green

| | | | Calories | | | | Calories |
|---|---|---|---|---|---|---|---|
| ¼ | cup | Broccoli | 11 | 1 | whole | Green pepper | 15 |
| 1 | cup | Spinach | 15 | ¼ | cup | Swiss chard | 14 |
| 1 | cup | Romaine | 10 | ¼ | cup | Mustard greens | 7.5 |
| 1 | bunch | Watercress | 17 | 4 | spears | Asparagus | 10 |
| ¼ | cup | Kale | 11 | ¼ | cup | Beet greens | 6 |
| ¼ | cup | Collard greens | 16 | | | | |

*2 Servings Per Day*

### Vegetables—Yellow and Other

| | | | | | | | |
|---|---|---|---|---|---|---|---|
| 1 | ear | Corn | 74 | 1 | medium | Onion | 26 |
| 1 | large | Carrot | 40 | 1 | cup | Boston or Bibb lettuce | 8 |
| ¼ | cup | Winter squash | 26 | ¼ | cup | Mung bean sprouts | 8 |
| 1 | cup | Pumpkin | 80 | ¼ | cup | Soybean sprouts | 18 |
| 1 | medium | Potato | 100 | 1 | | Artichoke | 85 |
| 1 | | Tomato | 25 | ¼ | cup | String beans | 9 |
| ¼ | cup | Beets | 18 | 1 | medium | Cucumber | 20 |
| ¼ | cup | Cauliflower | 8 | ¼ | cup | Zucchini | 7.5 |
| ¼ | cup | Cabbage | 5 | 1 | clove | Garlic | 6 |
| 1 | stalk | Celery | 8 | 1 | | Radish | 2 |
| 1 | large | Mushroom | 3 | | | | |

*1 Serving Per Day*

### Fruit

| | | | | | | | |
|---|---|---|---|---|---|---|---|
| 1 | medium | Apple | 80 | 1 | cup | Pineapple | 81 |
| 1 | medium | Banana | 100 | 1 | thick slice | Watermelon | 110 |
| 1 | medium | Pear | 100 | 1 | medium | Orange | 65 |
| 1 | medium | Apricot | 18 | ½ | | Grapefruit | 45 |
| 1 | wedge | Honeydew | 33 | 1 | 8-oz. glass | Fresh orange juice | 110 |
| ¼ | small | Cantaloupe | 36 | 1 | 8-oz. glass | Fresh grapefruit juice | 95 |
| ¼ | cup | Raspberries | 18 | | | | |
| ¼ | cup | Strawberries | 14 | 1 | 8-oz. glass | Unsweetened apple juice | 117 |
| ¼ | cup | Blueberries | 18 | 1 | whole | Kiwi | 46 |
| 1 | medium | Mango | 133 | 1 | whole | Plum | 30 |
| 1 | medium | Peach | 51 | 1 | small box | Raisins | 40 |
| 1 | medium | Papaya | 43 | | | | |

*2 Servings Per Day (if only one, choose a citrus)*

### Cereals, Breads, Grains

| | | | | | | | |
|---|---|---|---|---|---|---|---|
| 1 | slice | Whole-wheat bread (preferably stone ground) | 60 | 1 | cup | Puffed Corn (no salt/sugar) | 50 |
| ½ | cup | Oatmeal (non-instant) | 66 | ⅔ | cup | Cooked, long-grain brown rice | 133 |
| ½ | cup | Wheatena (non-instant) | 67 | 1 | cup | Parboiled (converted) white rice | 185 |
| ½ | cup | Cream of Wheat (non-instant) | 66 | ⅔ | cup | NutriGrain, corn | 110 |
| 1 | biscuit | Shredded Wheat | 89 | ½ | cup | Puffed Rice | 39 |
| ½ | cup | Spoon Size Shredded Wheat | 82 | ½ | cup | Puffed Wheat | 27 |
| | | | | 1 | cup | Rice Krispies | 110 |
| 1 | tablespoon | Wheat germ | 25 | 1 | cup | Cheerios | 110 |
| 1 | tablespoon | Yeast (brewer's) | 20 | ½ | cup | Cooked barley | 115 |
| ½ | cup | Cooked cornmeal (degermed) | 60 | ¼ | cup | Cooked spaghetti | 54 |
| 2 | cups | Air-popped popcorn | 46 | ¼ | cup | Cooked kasha (buckwheat groats) | 86 |
| 1 | | Corn tortilla | 111 | 1 | | Rice cake, unsalted | 34 |

*2 Servings Per Day*

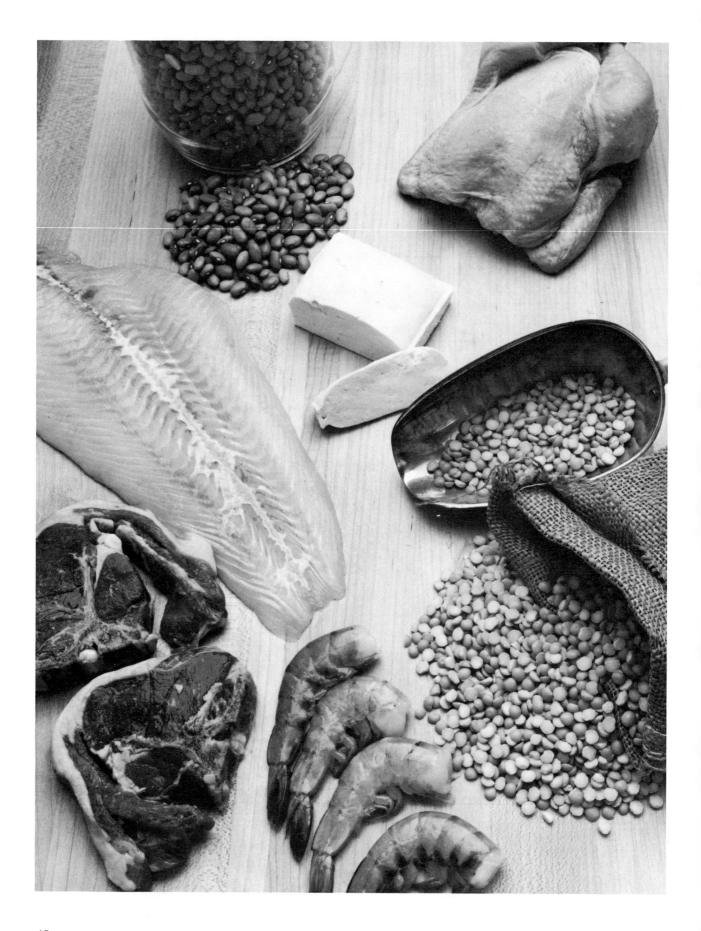

# Proteins

| | | | Calories |
|---|---|---|---|
| 1 | | Egg—boiled or poached (no more than 2 per week) | 80 |
| 2 | cups | My Protein Shake † (1 Tbs. protein powder/ unsweetened apple juice) | 174 |
| | | (3 Tbs. protein powder/nonfat milk) | 282 |

**1 Serving Per Day**

### Fish

| | | | |
|---|---|---|---|
| 3 | oz. | Abalone | 69 |
| 3 | oz. | Cod | 138 |
| 3 | oz. | Haddock | 121 |
| 3 | oz. | Sea bass | 82 |
| 3 | oz. | Halibut | 111 |
| 3 | oz. | Water-packed tuna | 100 |
| 3 | oz. | Flounder | 120 |
| 3 | oz. | Red snapper | 79 |
| 3 | oz. | Sole | 145 |
| 3 | oz. | Swordfish | 149 |

### Shellfish

| | | | |
|---|---|---|---|
| ½ | cup | Crab | 105 |
| ½ | cup | Shrimp | 103 |
| ½ | cup | Crayfish | 82 |

### Poultry

| | | | |
|---|---|---|---|
| 3 | oz. | White-meat turkey without skin | 150 |
| | | skin punctured to drain fat | 190 |
| 3 | oz. | White-meat chicken without skin (Fryer has less fat than roasting chicken) | 142 |
| 3 | oz. | Cornish hen | 150 |

### Beans*

**1 Serving Per Day**

| | | | |
|---|---|---|---|
| ½ | cup | Cooked lentils | 106 |
| ½ | cup | Cooked kidney beans | 109 |
| ½ | cup | Cooked split peas | 115 |
| ½ | cup | medium or firm tofu | 90 |

(Tofu is bland, firm, and custardlike. It is made from curdled soy milk and is very low in calories and high in protein. I use it in salads, dips, and soups, scramble it in eggs, add it to stews and casseroles)

### Beef (these are the leaner cuts)

**1 Serving Once or Twice a Week**

| | | | |
|---|---|---|---|
| 3 | oz. | Roast beef (round) | 160 |
| 3 | oz. | London broil (hind-shank) | 155 |
| 3 | oz. | Pot roast (fore-shank) | 165 |
| 3 | oz. | Flank steak (wedge or round bone) | 166.5 |
| 3 | oz. | Sirloin (wedge or round bone) | 175 |
| 3 | oz. | Hamburger | |
| | | lean | 185 |
| | | regular | 245 |

### Lamb

**1 Serving Once or Twice a Week**

| | | | |
|---|---|---|---|
| 3 | oz. | Leg of lamb | 150 |
| 3 | oz. | Loin chop | 122 |

### Veal

| | | | |
|---|---|---|---|
| 3 | oz. | Leg (foreshank) | 159 |
| 3 | oz. | Loin chop | 176 |

*NOTE: Please see the chart on page 34, which will guide you in getting complete protein from beans, as well as in combining other complementary foods, in order to lessen your dependency on meats for protein.

†Recipe on page 53.

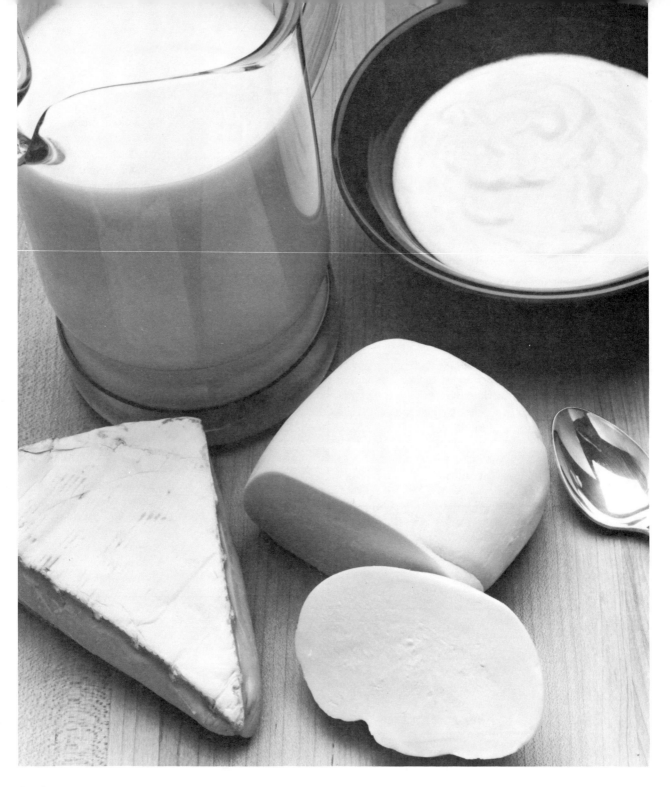

# Dairy

| | | | | Calories | | | Calories |
|---|---|---|---|---|---|---|---|
| **2 Servings Per Day** | 1 | cup | 1% low-fat milk | 100 | 1¼ oz. | Mozzarella | 80 |
| | 1 | cup | Buttermilk | 100 | 1¼ oz. | Farmer cheese | 125 |
| | 1 | cup | Nonfat milk | 85 | 1¼ oz. | Feta | 95 |
| | 1 | cup | Low-fat plain yogurt | 145 | 1¼ oz. | Neufchâtel | 91 |
| | 1 | cup | Low-fat cottage cheese | 165 | 2 oz. | Camembert | 170 |

## Fats

| 1 Choice Per Day | | | | *Calories* |
|---|---|---|---|---|
| | 1 | tablespoon | Corn oil | 120 |
| | 1 | tablespoon | Safflower oil | 120 |
| | 1 | tablespoon | Sesame oil | 120 |
| | 1 | tablespoon | Olive oil | 120 |

Safflower has little taste. Sesame has a nutty flavor; you'll probably want to use only a few drops for flavor. Corn oil has a buttery flavor.

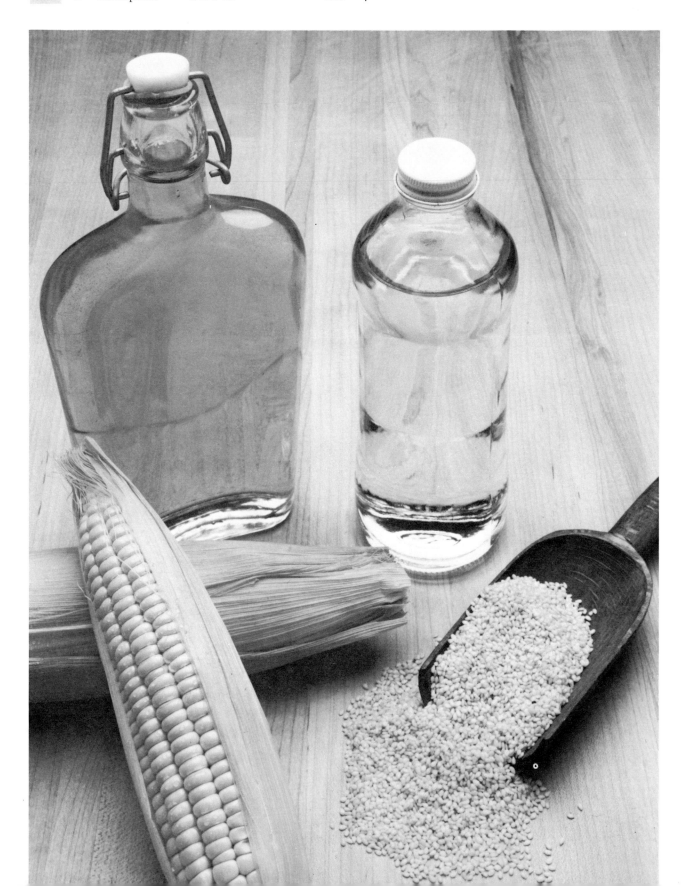

## A MEAL-BY-MEAL OVERVIEW

### Breakfast:

Don't skip *breakfast!* Breakfast sets you up and gives you energy for the day. Several studies have shown that eating breakfast regularly may be a factor in a longer life. It will certainly allow you to feel satisfied until lunch and untempted to grab for a sweet roll as a pick-me-up.

But *what* you eat for breakfast is critical. This meal should include fresh fruit, either whole or as juice. Remember, one-half grapefruit (75 calories) or a medium orange (65 calories) has fewer calories and more fiber than an 8-ounce glass of fresh orange juice (110 calories) or grapefruit juice (95 calories).

The breakfast meal should definitely include some other complex carbohydrate, preferably whole-grain cereal or bread. The dry cereals recom-

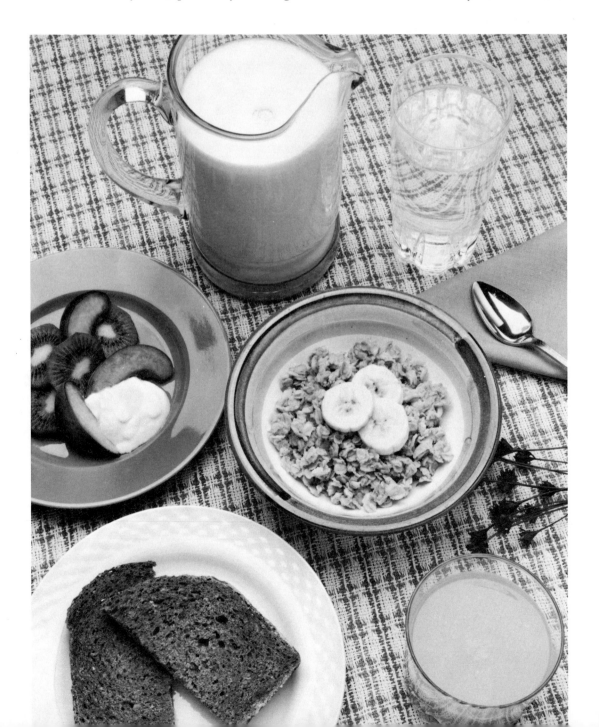

mended for a weight-loss diet are listed on page 47. Preferably, cooked cereals should not be the instant varieties since the process used to make them "instant" reduces the nutrient value. Use nonfat milk on the cereal, and instead of sugar get into the habit of using berries or sliced fruit like bananas or apples as a sweetener. The whole-wheat (preferably stone-ground) bread or toast should not be buttered. Unsweetened apple butter is nice if you have trouble getting used to dry toast. (By the way, toast has the same number of calories as untoasted bread.) As you wean yourself away from using sugar on your cereal and butter on your toast, your taste buds will become more sensitized to subtler tastes. The complex flavor and texture of whole wheats and grains will prove very satisfying. Chew slowly and savor these treats.

I'm especially fond of hot Irish oatmeal in the morning. It's crunchier and chewier than rolled oats. When I'm traveling, oatmeal is my favorite low-calorie room-service breakfast. I ask for it to be cooked with no salt or sugar and served with nonfat milk instead of cream. Actually, I go back a ways with oatmeal. When I was around ten years old, I took an exam I had been worried about and did very well. Before going to school that morning, I had eaten oatmeal for breakfast and came to associate it with my success on the test. From then on, I had oatmeal before every exam (it didn't always work!) and began to call it "brain food." Now, of course, I realize that my childhood intuition was quite on target. It is now known that a hearty breakfast of complex carbohydrates like oatmeal increases a person's attention span, ability to concentrate, and ability to think clearly.

In addition to your carbohydrates, be sure to get some breakfast protein. This can be the milk on your cereal or some yogurt with your fruit. If you're at home and have a blender, you might concoct a protein drink for breakfast. Here's my recipe below.

Eggs are another source of protein, but I recommend no more than two eggs a week. The yolks contain very high levels of cholesterol. The best way to serve them is boiled in their shell or poached on your whole-wheat toast.

---

### MY PROTEIN SHAKE

Combine the following in a blender:
   1 cup nonfat milk or unsweetened apple juice (or a combination of both—the apple juice is the sweetener)
   3 or 4 fresh or fresh-frozen strawberries (or ⅓ cup blueberries or peaches—never with syrup!)
   1 half of a fresh banana
   1 tablespoon nonfat plain yogurt
   1 to 3 tablespoons protein powder
      (preferably made from milk and egg protein with no sugar, artificial coloring, or flavor added)
      A few ice cubes, if fruit isn't frozen.
Blend for one minute.

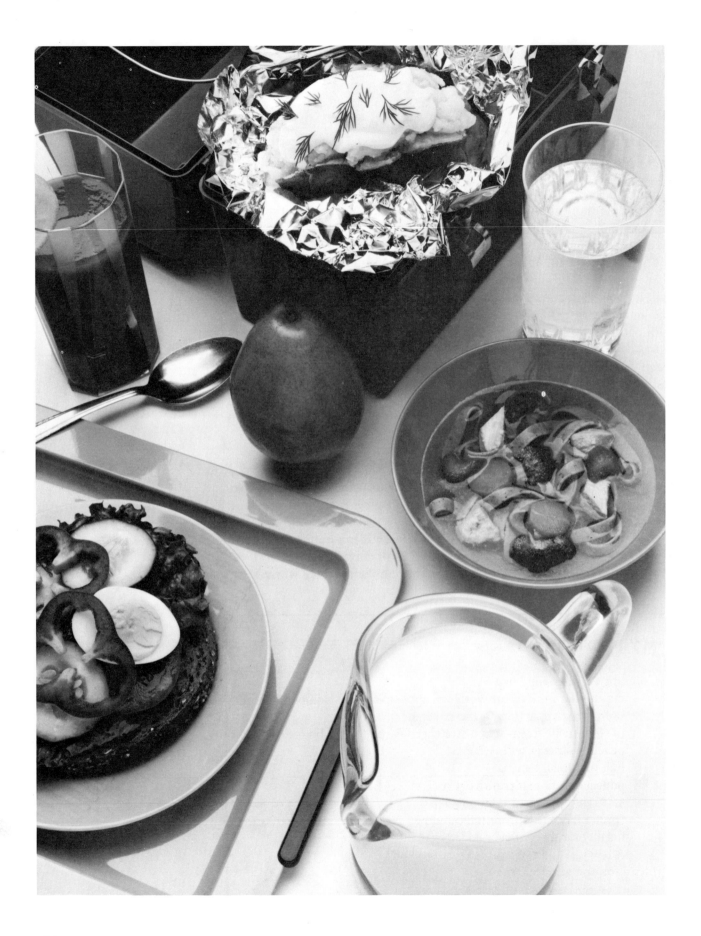

## Lunch:

Lunch is a good time to emphasize protein as well as carbohydrates. The protein can be cottage cheese, yogurt, a small portion of skinless white meat of chicken or turkey, fish, or a hardboiled egg. Your carbohydrates can be raw or cooked vegetables in a salad. Try making an open-faced sandwich using your choices from the list with one nice thick slice of whole-wheat bread (try it on stone-ground and sprouted wheat bread).

Soup is an excellent way to have a filling, satisfying lunch that fills both your protein and carbohydrate requirements. In fact, soup should be a regular part of your weight-loss diet. It's generally lower in calories than solid foods, assuming it's been de-fatted and made without cream or butter. We tend to eat soup slowly because it's hot, but it enters the bloodstream quickly so it speedily triggers the mechanism that lets us know we've had enough. You'll feel more satiated before you've had time to consume a lot of calories. If you want to thicken your soups, try using low-fat milk or a puree of the soup's vegetables.

If you don't have access to a cafeteria that has a good salad bar with a wide variety of fresh vegetables, then make a habit of brown-bagging it. The time you save not going to a restaurant, with the waiting and the lines, might give you a chance to do a workout or to go for a jog or walk.

For the best never-feel-deprived brown-bag lunches, you'll need a wide-mouthed thermos for soup, cooked protein, or whatever pasta or grain you may have cooked. You'll need a plastic container for salad ingredients or sandwich filling. I advise bringing your slice of bread separately so you can make the sandwich fresh. (That way, it doesn't get soggy.) Finally, you'll need a container for your low-calorie salad dressing.

I often bring a baked potato with me for lunch. I eat it at room temperature plain or with the following topping:

---

### COTTAGE CREAM

I found this excellent recipe in *Jane Brody's Good Food Book.*\* This is a good substitute for sour cream, especially as a topping on baked potatoes.

    3 tablespoons milk or buttermilk
    1 tablespoon lemon juice
    1 cup low-fat cottage cheese

1. In a blender combine the milk and lemon juice. With the blender on low speed, gradually add the cottage cheese. Increase the speed to high, and blend the mixture for about 2 minutes.
2. Transfer the cream to a jar, cover it, and refrigerate it. If the cream becomes too thick, thin it by stirring in a little milk or buttermilk.

\* *Jane Brody's Good Food Book,* by Jane Brody (W. W. Norton, 1985).

---

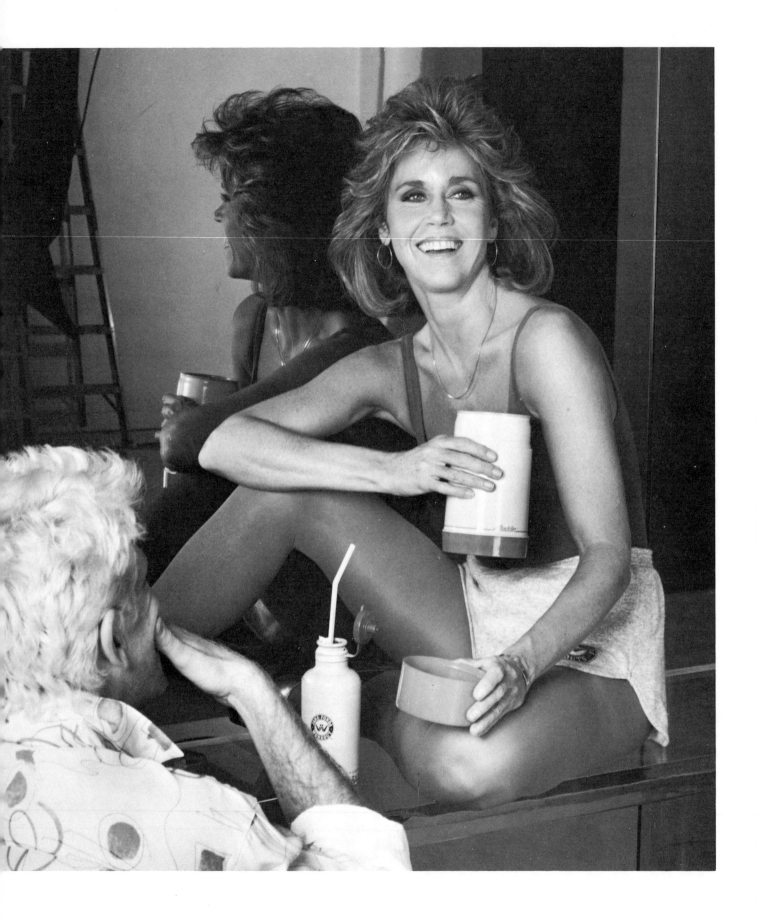

Forget about cold cuts, luncheon meats, pickles, and the like. These are some of the salty, fatty, calorie-dense, nutrient-poor ingredients you're training yourself to do without. You can include a small piece of fruit or unsweetened applesauce with low-fat plain yogurt, if you like, for a satisfying lunchtime dessert.

I advise against having a fruit salad as your main lunch course, however. Such a concentration of sugar, even though it is complex, will give you a quick energy jolt, but tend to drop you down along about midafternoon. If a fruit salad is the only healthy choice offered you, have it with some protein such as low-fat cottage cheese or low-fat plain yogurt.

## Snacks:

Many nutritionists report the benefits of eating a number of small meals throughout the day rather than one or two big ones. Like me, I'm sure you know women who starve all day and then eat a big dinner; maybe you're one of them. If so, please understand how counterproductive that is. Having only a few large meals, it appears, encourages fat storage, erratic mood-swings, and even the risk of heart disease. These problems are especially acute when the big meal is eaten late at night. All this argues in favor of having a nutritious snack during the afternoon around 3:00 P.M. or 4:00 P.M. This is the time when most of us begin to feel our energy flagging. Such a snack is especially important if our largest meal comes toward the end of the day.

Here are some suggestions for this snack:

One-half banana
One small carrot
Two stalks celery
One small cucumber
A hunk of raw cabbage (with or without a low-calorie dressing)
One-half cup of dry, unsalted *air-popped* popcorn
Two saltless rice cakes
One bran wafer
One-half baked potato
One endive
Four ounces salt-free tomato juice
Four ounces unsweetened apple juice
One medium apple
Four ounces low-fat yogurt with a small piece of fruit

Because you are restricting your caloric intake, what you choose will depend on what you have already eaten and what you plan to eat for dinner. Look at the calorie count in your list of recommended foods on pages 47–51 to make your determination.

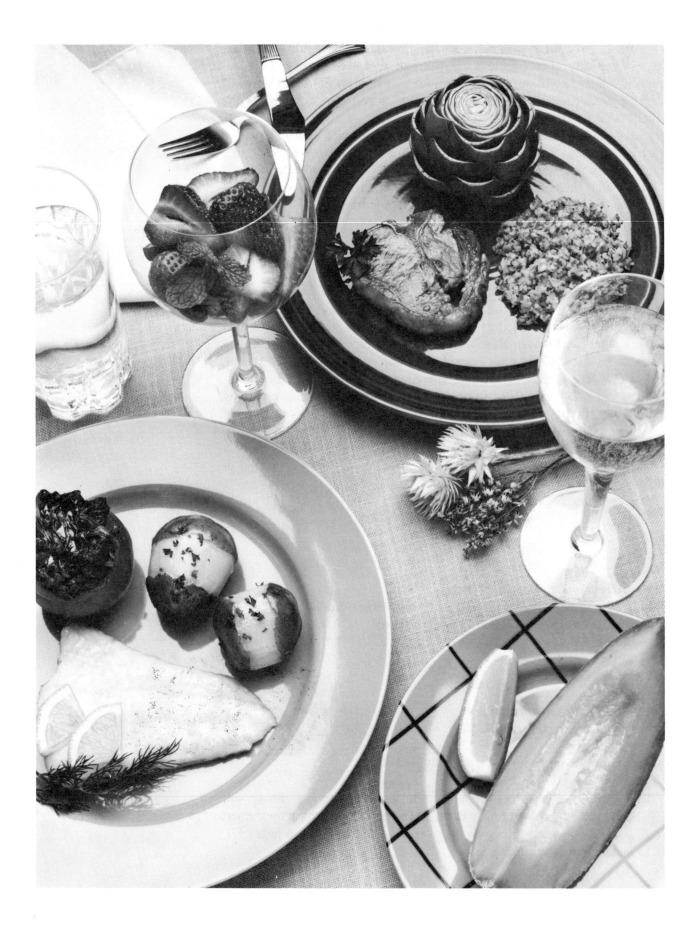

## Dinner:

Try not to eat dinner much after 7:00 P.M., if at all possible. In one well-publicized study, a group of people were fed one 2,000-calorie meal a day, either as breakfast, lunch, or dinner. Those who ate all these calories for breakfast *lost* weight, those who ate them for lunch *maintained* their weight, and those who saved them for dinner *gained*. The time of day made a difference of up to two and one-half pounds!

Your dinner meal should stress carbohydrates because they release the brain chemical serotonin, which helps you sleep. Use proteins such as fish, poultry (without skin), or lean meat in very small amounts as a condiment to accompany your starch, such as rice, pasta, or potatoes. As I said earlier, although we're used to thinking of the starches as fattening, they're not. It's what we put on them that kills us. There are many excellent cookbooks available now with healthy, low-calorie, low-fat, but *delicious* recipes. My new favorite is *Jane Brody's Good Food Book.*

If you're eating alone or with family, hot soup with a slice of bread and a vegetable or salad is an ideal dinner.

---

### TOMATO SALAD DRESSING*

This is my adaptation of a recipe for salad dressing in *Diet for Life:*

- ⅔ cup tomato juice, no salt added
- ¼ cup corn oil
- 1 tablespoon apple-cider vinegar
- 2 tablespoons fresh lemon juice
- ½ teaspoon ground ginger
- 2 shallots, finely minced
- 4 dashes cayenne pepper
- 1 teaspoon each minced fresh tarragon and parsley
- 2 tablespoons unsweetened apple juice

1. Combine all ingredients in jar, and shake well. Let stand for one hour before using. Shake again before serving.
2. This dressing will keep well, refrigerated, for four days. Remove from refrigerator an hour before serving. Yield: 1 cup

* from *Diet for Life,* by Francine Prince. (New York: Cornerstone, 1981).

---

## TOMATO-HERB DRESSING*

  6 ounces (1 small can) tomato juice or V-8
  ¼ cup apple-cider vinegar
  2 tablespoons olive oil
  1 tablespoon fresh lemon juice
  1 tablespoon Dijon mustard
  1 tablespoon fresh chopped chives
  1 tablespoon fresh minced parsley
  1 large clove garlic, crushed
  ½ teaspoon dried basil or 1 tablespoon fresh minced basil
  ⅛ teaspoon cayenne, or to taste

In a bowl or jar, combine all the dressing ingredients, whisking or shaking them to blend them well.

(*Variation:* For a thicker dressing, try adding about 4 ounces of tofu (soybean curd), creaming the ingredients together in a blender or food processor. This would increase the yield to about 2 cups.)

* (from *Jane Brody's Good Food Book*)

## COOKING VEGETABLES

1. Don't overcook vegetables or allow them to soak in water.
2. Don't cut them up until just before cooking.
3. Steaming or microwaving is infinitely better than boiling.
4. When you do boil, save the vegetable cooking water for stocks and soups.

### Eating Out:

If you're going out to eat, try having a glass of water and a light snack before you leave. Carrot sticks, celery, half an apple, or an unsalted rice cake can take the edge off your hunger and make you less apt to overeat.

Don't feel self-conscious about telling your waiter that you don't want your food cooked with butter, salt, or MSG. Good restaurants have grown accustomed to these requests and are usually prepared to serve lighter, low-fat meals. Ask for your vegetables to be steamed al dente (still firm to the bite) and for your salad to be brought with no dressing or with the dressing on the side. Here's a quick dressing you can make yourself at the table:

Ask for lemon juice or vinegar and Dijon mustard. Mix them together to taste with a dash of Sweet 'n Low. (My one concession to a sugar substitute.)

One warning: Don't make a big deal of any of this. There's nothing worse than eating with someone who goes on and on about his or her diet. It's perfectly possible to get what you want gracefully and quietly. The others at your table will appreciate it and may be better motivated (because not guilt-tripped) to follow your example.

You can make the same kind of choices when you take a plane trip. If you call at least twenty-four hours in advance, you can have a low-fat, lower-calorie, or vegetarian meal. Alcohol is definitely ill-advised while flying. It contributes to the dehydration that occurs on flights and exacerbates jet lag. The best way to avoid or minimize jet lag is to drink lots of water, eat little, and avoid alcohol.

Speaking of drinks, let's discuss them awhile.

## Drinks:

*Alcohol.* Besides its addictive dangers, alcohol is full of calories, *empty* calories. For someone on a weight-loss program I recommend eliminating alcohol or cutting down to the barest minimum. Remember, alcohol increases your appetite and reduces your willpower. If you have wine with your meal, you might try diluting it with club soda or sparkling mineral water. This allows you to extend one glass of wine through the whole meal, although admittedly it alters the unique bouquet and flavor of the wine.

COMPARE THE CALORIES

|  | *calories per gram* |
|---|---|
| Fats | 9 |
| *Alcohol* | 7 |
| Protein | 4 |
| Carbohydrates | 4 |

*Fruit Juices.* Your fruit juices should always be unsweetened (never nectars). Try diluting juices with club sodas or mineral water.

*Water.* Water is one of the most essential elements of any weight-loss diet. When feeling sluggish, we often reach for food when there's a good chance we're dehydrated and what our body really needs is water. Drinking caffeine and alcohol can dehydrate us, as can drinking too little water. Try to drink six to eight glasses a day. Don't wait until you're parched with thirst. Drinking a glass before each meal is a good idea. It will help fill you up. (Water is also a natural diuretic that helps flush water-retaining sodium out of the body.)

## Desserts:

I know it's hard but I want to encourage you to wean yourself away from your sweet tooth. This means not relying on artificial sweeteners, which just maintain your addiction to sweet tastes and never helped anyone lose weight. From time to time, if you do have dessert, choose fruit ices and

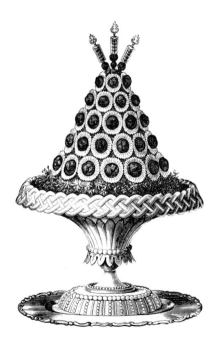

sorbets that contain no fat, or frozen yogurt sherbets, which have less fat and fewer calories than regular ice cream. Chilled fresh fruit is a fine way to finish a meal sweetly.

## 10 TIPS TO REMEMBER

1. Establish *regular eating habits:* three—or more—meals a day at routine intervals, composed of a healthy variety of foods, including solid fibrous foods you must chew.
2. Don't skip meals, especially breakfast.
3. Carry some raw vegetables or a piece of fruit with you as an afternoon pick-me-up for that hour when blood sugar levels tend to drop and you're tempted to reach for sweets.
4. Don't chew gum. It stimulates the salivary glands and makes you feel hungry when you otherwise wouldn't.
5. Try not to shop when you're hungry.
6. Don't eat absent-mindedly while talking on the phone, reading, or watching TV.
7. Eat slowly and chew well so your digestive enzymes begin to work *before* food reaches the stomach. Your food will then have time to be absorbed into the blood and trigger the "had enough" signal before you've overeaten. By eating fast you fill your stomach with more food than you may need to satisfy your *true* physical needs.
8. Eat sitting down.
9. Take time to savor and enjoy what you are eating.
10. If you feel a binge coming on, take a fast walk, an hour-long one, if possible. Your hunger will cool down as your body heats up.

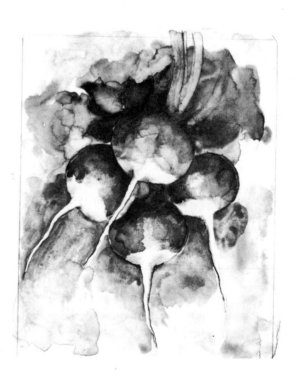

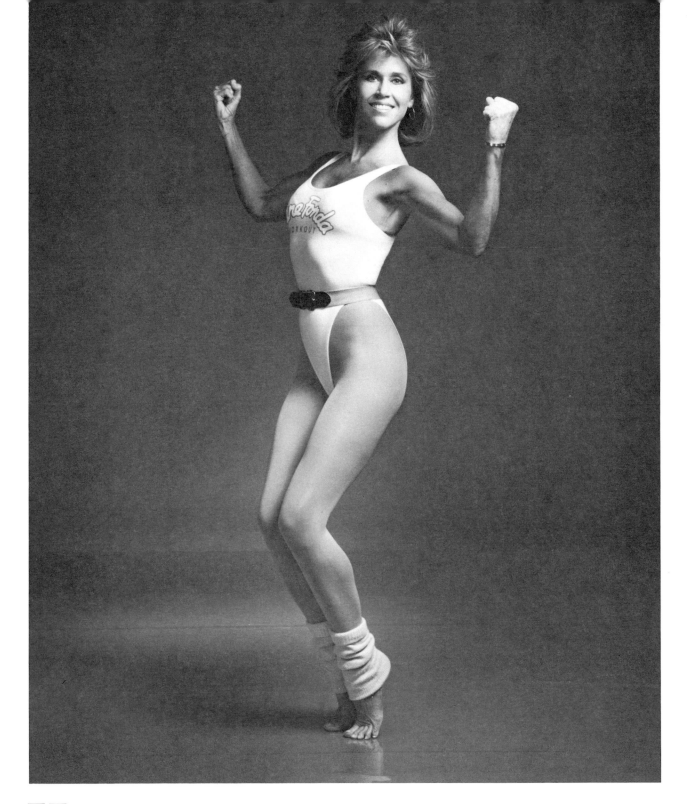

# II · THE EXERCISE
# COMPONENT

# EXERCISE AND WEIGHT LOSS

Now that you're familiar with the nutritional basics, you might ask, wouldn't it be possible for you to just diet in order to lose weight? Yes, it would. But there are two major drawbacks to this approach: Weight loss through dieting alone is mainly temporary. It is also very, very difficult.

Weight loss occurs when your caloric intake is less than what you burn up in the course of a day. If you rely solely on reducing food intake, your diet is going to have to be much more restrictive and hence harder to stick to than if you combine a less restrictive, well-balanced diet with increased energy output. For instance, if the only thing you changed in your life was to walk for an hour every day for a year—without changing the number of calories you consumed—you could lose 30 pounds. There's no question about it; for permanent body-fat weight loss, diet plus exercise is the answer.

In addition to the important benefit of burning calories, there are other more long-lasting effects of exercise. Certain processes are set in motion by exercise that have an even greater influence on weight control.

- First of all, it's essential to understand the central role of aerobic exercise in losing weight. It's important for burning calories, of course, but it's specifically important for burning *fat* calories. Aerobic exercise requires a lot of fuel and favors stored fat as its fuel source. It uses the quick-energy supply of glucose to get the body moving in the first minutes of exercise, but then it turns to the body's fat supply, a more plentiful and denser fuel that needs a lot of oxygen in order to be burned. (Aerobics, by definition, means exercising "with oxygen.") Aerobic exercise is the only safe and effective way to mobilize subcutaneous fat from *all over* the body. It also gets to the marbled fat *deep inside the muscle*—one of the things dieting alone *can't* do.
- As your aerobic fitness increases through regular, strenuous (but not excessive) exercise, your basal metabolic rate increases too. The body becomes more efficient at utilizing calories as energy all through the day. It also becomes less disposed to storing fat and more inclined to burn calories for energy even when resting.
- The metabolism is tuned up not only by aerobic exercise, but also by exercises that specifically work the muscle groups of the whole body, like those given at the Workout and in weight-training programs. All of these maintain or increase your active muscle tissue. In this way, exercise improves your metabolism while ensuring that your weight loss is from fat and not from muscle. At minimum, exercise acts as a muscle preservative.
- Exercise decreases your appetite, especially if you exercise an hour or so before a meal. Normally, you feel hungry when your blood sugar level

drops. But when you exercise regularly, your blood sugar level remains more stable. This is because your muscles are using proportionately more fat than sugar as fuel. And there is also less insulin in the blood, which otherwise would act to lower blood sugar levels.

• Exercise creates more of the special enzymes that break down stored fat into fatty acids and transfer them to the metabolically active muscle tissue where they are burned as energy.

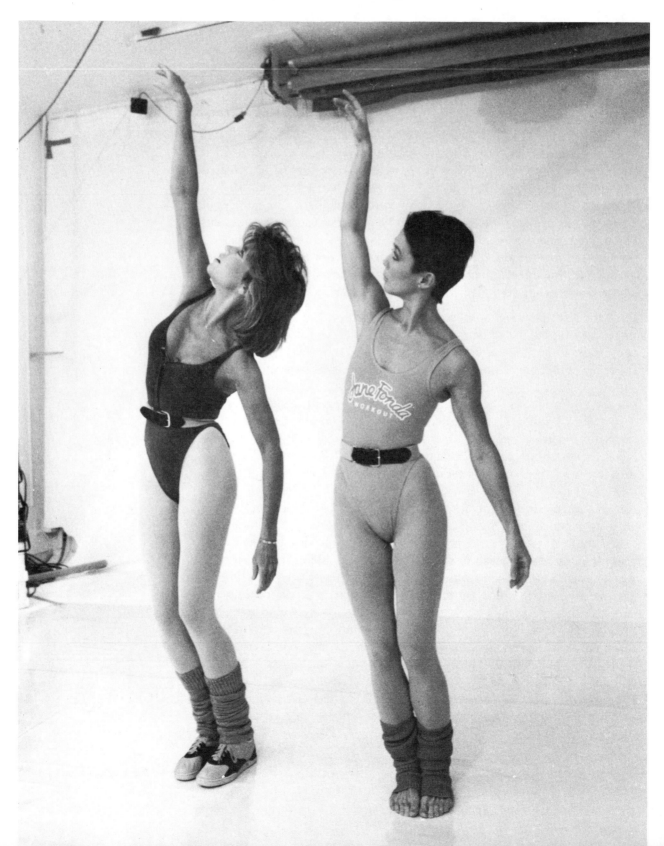

# GUIDELINES

The exercise guidelines that follow are meant to go hand-in-glove with the dieting guidelines.

1. Compulsive exercise is as unhealthful as compulsive eating. Seek balance and moderation in both.
2. Exercise aerobically at least three times a week, *preferably* four or five times, but no more than six days a week. The body needs at least one day to rest and repair itself.
3. Exercise aerobically for at least 30 minutes—45 to 60 minutes is ideal if your schedule permits. (Beginners, please be sure to start slowly, at your own level, and build up gradually.) Each session should burn between 300 to 500 calories. Three miles walked briskly or jogged, for instance, will burn about 300 calories (of course, walking will require a little more time than jogging to cover the same distance).
4. Exercise within your aerobic training range. (See box on page 78 for how to calculate yours.) In the beginning, the pulse is your best and most convenient check. Whether you can carry on a conversation without becoming excessively breathless while exercising is another. Remember, you want to be drinking in oxygen, so the exercise can't be so fast you're gasping for air and have to quit after a short burst of effort. If that happens, you'll know you're exercising *an*aerobically, that is, without oxygen, and without mobilizing fat stores. On the other hand, the effort can't be so easy you don't call upon the cardiorespiratory system to improve. The goal is lots of oxygen for a sustained period.

Just think. There are 3,500 calories in one fat pound. If you combine *burning 500 calories more* with *eating 500 calories less,* you'll have a deficit of 1,000 calories at the day's end and *two pounds* at the week's end—and nearly all in fat!

## THE ROLE OF PATIENCE

What if you've been exercising vigorously and following your diet carefully, but the pounds just aren't coming off? Or what if you've lost weight, but are now on a weight plateau that has stayed the same for weeks? Be patient. Each body responds differently. Each body, and mind, begins the diet in a different state of fitness. Eventually, with calm persistence, the fat melts away.

*pposite: **Demonstrating a stretch to Diane Toyama Ekker.***

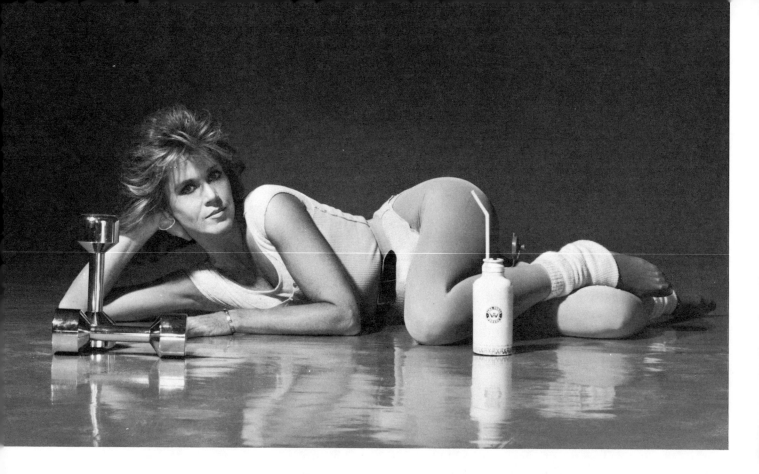

There are a number of reasons why weight loss may be slower than expected. As you begin to burn up fat for muscle fuel, for instance, your body tends to retain water. This water weight will not be permanent; the excess fluid will eventually be eliminated as sweat and urine. You also have to remember that muscle weighs more than fat and takes up less space. You will probably find that you lose inches before you start losing pounds. The secret to losing weight is patience, regular vigorous *but not excessive* exercise, and the determination to push yourself, gently, beyond what you were able to do yesterday.

Don't forget that the longer you stick to the diet and the more consistently and gradually you lose weight, the more your weight loss will represent lost body fat.

Once you lose the fat pounds you wanted to lose, once you achieve the weight that's best for you, you can begin to consciously restore to your diet the calories you subtracted during the time you were dieting. You can do this by eating larger portions, or more of the higher-caloried complex carbohydrates. You can have more fruit, for instance, more bread, more nuts.

Once you've followed this diet, you possess the fundamentals of what can be a lifelong way of eating. If you continue to exercise regularly, you've got a solid program you can really count on to keep you fit, lean, and feeling good.

# GETTING SERIOUS

I wish that I could tell you that exercising regularly is easy. It's not. In fact, I think that for most people the hardest part of exercising is getting yourself on a program. It takes determination, commitment, and discipline. When people tell me they just can't seem to get started, I'm reminded of my experience with Katharine Hepburn. I've told the story of my "Golden Pond back flip" in my first book but I think it bears repeating.

My role in *On Golden Pond* called for my character to do a back flip into the chilly waters of Squam Lake in New Hampshire. As I'd never done a back dive before, much less a back flip, I figured that a stunt woman could easily fill in for me in that scene. As a childhood klutz and a Californian who hates cold water, why should I willingly fling myself backwards into a freezing lake?

Then I met Miss Hepburn. She wondered if I would be doing the back flip myself and let it be known that *she* could do one. I found out that she had been a competitive diver at one time, and then I remembered that great dive she made in *Philadelphia Story.* I felt challenged, and I must confess that I

*Katharine Hepburn doing a high kick in* On Golden Pond

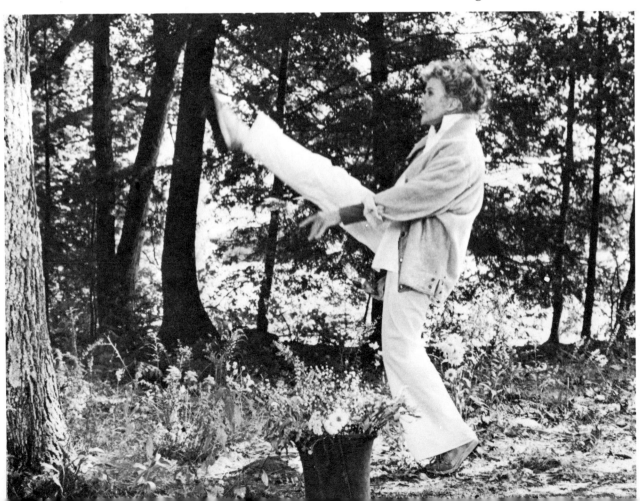

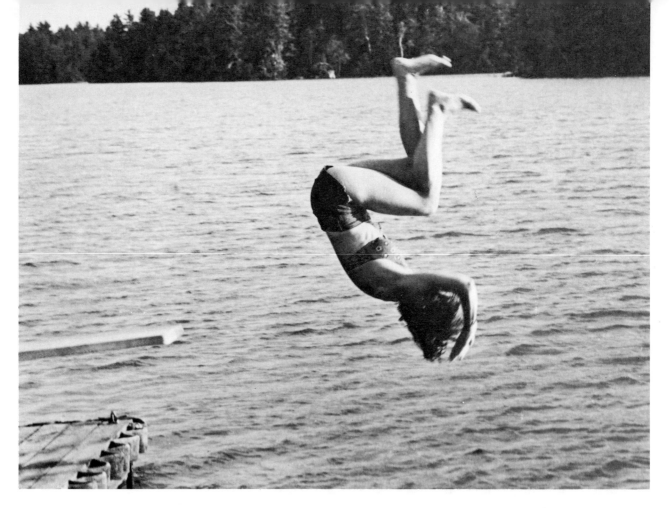

wanted her to like me, so I decided I would try my best to learn to do a back flip.

Day after day that summer I practiced with a terrific instructor, first in a pool and then from a float in Squam Lake. I was awful. My legs would slam against the water so hard they were red and bruised. All my adolescent convictions about being a klutz came back in waves. It got so that I was terrified every time I tried that flip, but I did not want to lose Miss Hepburn's respect, so I kept going.

Finally I mastered it. Nothing to write home about, but it was a back flip, and I could do it. One day as I was climbing out of that icy water, Miss Hepburn approached me. "Don't you feel good?"

"Just terrific," I said. And I did. Miss Hepburn must have recognized the way I felt because she said, "Everyone should know that feeling of overcoming fear and mastering something. People who aren't taught that become soggy!"

Miss Hepburn is the least soggy person I know. That summer at Squam Lake she told me of the pleasure she has in extending herself physically. In her seventies she is a testament to non-sogginess. I certainly will be less soggy as a result of knowing her. She made me realize that it is never too late to master your weaknesses and feel the elation that comes with pushing yourself to new levels. You may be soggy today, but there is no reason for you to be soggy tomorrow.

If you are serious about wanting to get fit, about improving your self-image and your morale, you must kiss your sogginess good-bye. There are no shortcuts. No sweatless quickies. You must be committed to working hard, sweating hard, and getting a little sore. You cannot do it passively by going to a spa and having your bottom jiggled on a vibrating belt, taking a few swipes at bicycling, or sitting in a sauna. All you would be doing is fooling yourself and wasting your money.

You have to be determined, and you also have to be smart. If you expect more of yourself than you are capable of doing, for instance, all your well-intentioned exercise efforts can be counterproductive. The guilt you feel when you can't live up to your own unreasonable demands on yourself may send you right back to sagging spirits and soggy living. Endurance and strength are built up *gradually,* with a measure of passion, yes, but with a measure of patience as well. Please don't push yourself so hard that you burn out.

How do you get started? Wherever I go, this is the question I hear over and over. It's asked so often because getting a routine going is undeniably the hardest part. Even when there's motivation, there's always the problem of time. You have to shove other stuff aside, somehow, and pile exercise on top of what seems like an already burdensome schedule.

My answer to the list of obstacles is always the same. You have to *make* it happen. You have to fashion a solution for yourself, anticipating that it will probably be tough to implement in the beginning. I'm sure you know some

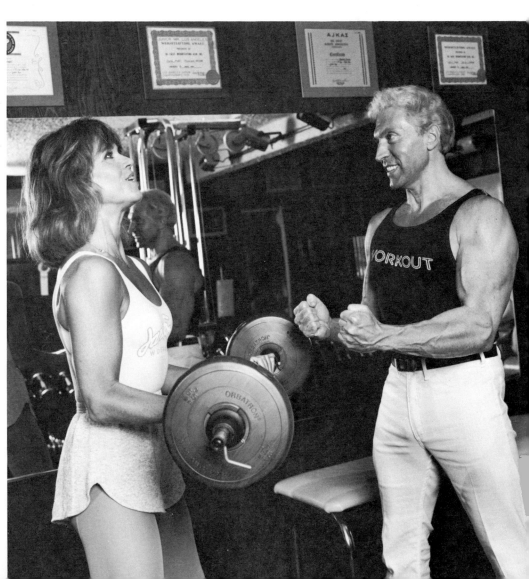

*Me with trainer, Dr. Bernie Ernst, co-star of the popular syndicated TV show* Body Buddies

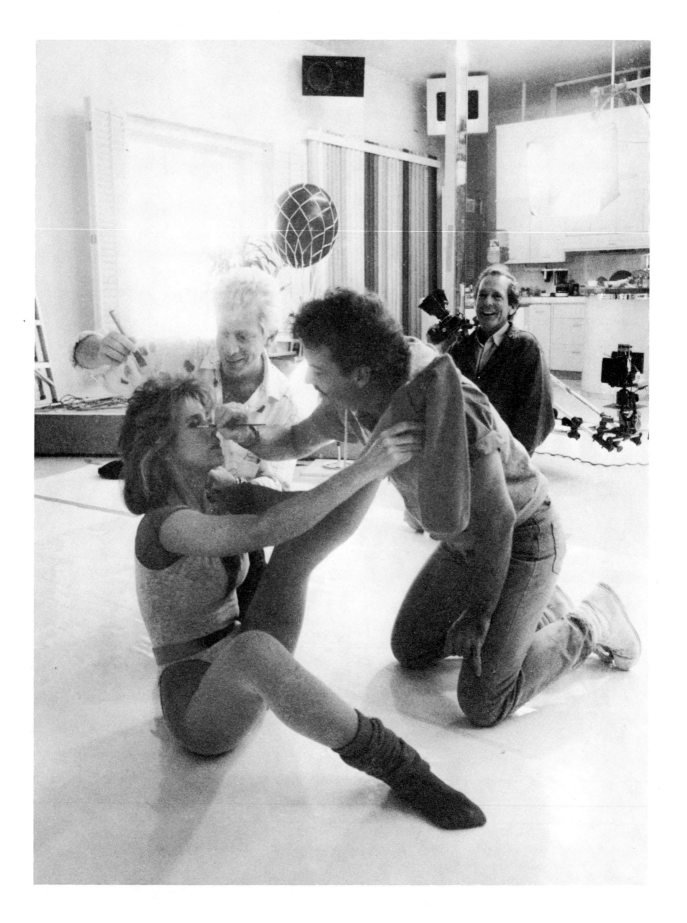

of the best strategies: getting up earlier, exchanging exercise for lunch (you can brown-bag it afterward), stopping at class or the gym on your way home from work, using the time when your kid is napping, or arranging with another family member to help with cooking three or four times a week so you can work out instead of preparing dinner. To make it easier, I've put my various Workouts onto audio and video tapes, so you can get the motivation that a class gives you even if you work out in your own home.

There's no reason why vigorous exercise cannot be a regular part of your life. I have a frantically busy schedule, with long erratic hours of work, plus children, a husband, a house to run—the works. But for the past twenty years, I've made sure I get a workout in four to six times a week. I've experienced its very real rewards. I simply schedule it into my life as if my life depends on it, which in a way it does. I do it for myself. And I do it no matter what.

It's not easy. Fitting three or four workouts into the week is hard at first. You will always have a good reason to skip one. You could be cleaning the house, running errands, baking, catching up on work, watching a movie, or sleeping late.

"How is it," you may ask, "that some people seem to be addicted to exercise when I can't even get started?" Well, it may be because regular exercisers have experienced the effects of certain natural compounds called endorphins and enkephalins that are produced in the body during a vigorous workout. These have an opiatelike effect, reducing depression and pain, increasing alertness and relaxation, and improving your mood and overall mental well-being. With all these positive by-products in addition to the calorie-burning, appetite-reducing effects of exercise, it's not so hard to see why more and more previously inactive women and men are overcoming its inconvenience and making their workout a permanent part of their lives.

Once *you* discipline yourself to exercise, once *you* experience the exhilaration afterward, once *you* become accustomed to the regular energy-rush and tension-release, you'll start to miss your workouts when you don't do them. Tough as it is to get yourself in gear, you'll always have that reward of feeling so much better at the other end.

*posite: **The wrecking crew at work***

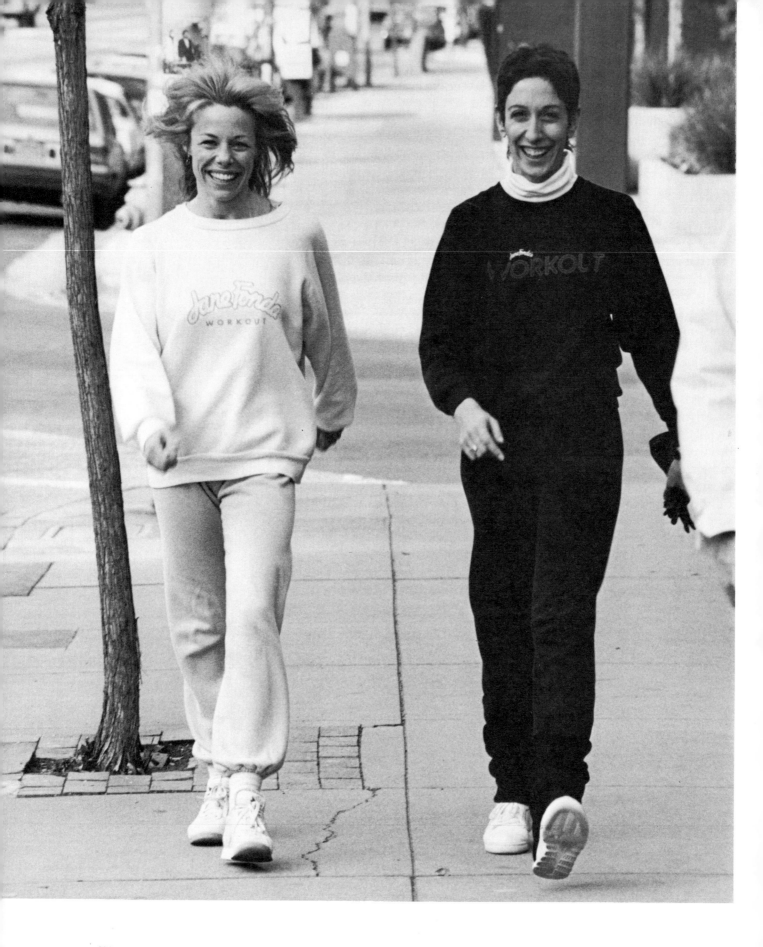

# SELECTING WHAT YOU DO

The kind of exercise you choose will depend in part on the facilities available to you: whether there is a track, jogging route, swimming pool, gym, or stimulating dance or exercise class in your neighborhood, or whether you have a stereo or video player in your home.

If you have any serious physical problem, I suggest you consult an exercise physiologist or sports medicine doctor. These can be located through a local sports medicine clinic or a university hospital which offers either a wellness program or preventive medicine, cardiac rehabilitation, or sports medicine programs. Experts in these areas can tell you what exercises you should and should not do.

The exercise program you set up for yourself should include aerobics for cardiovascular conditioning and endurance, resistance exercises to increase your muscle strength, and stretching for flexibility. My New Workout, which I outline in detail in Part III, fits my needs in all three areas, but everyone has her own temperament and body rhythm, so when you develop your own exercise program, listen to your body.

If you are going to stick with your workout program—and I think of mine as a lifetime commitment—it has to be something that suits you and that you enjoy. Enjoyable does not necessarily mean easy. The joy comes from accomplishing something you did not think you could do before.

But whatever type of workout you settle on, it should include the Big Three of health and fitness—aerobics, resistance exercises, and stretching.

## AEROBICS

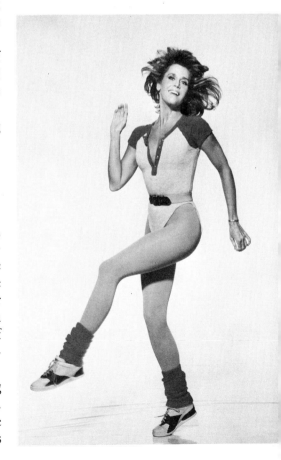

Aerobic exercise is the foundation of any fitness program. Aerobics are, literally, the heart of the matter. They improve and sustain the cardiorespiratory system, which is the key to the vitality of the entire body. They make us breathe deeply, sending a rich supply of oxygen through the blood to the muscles so the muscles can then produce energy. How much oxygen your lungs inhale, how much blood your heart pumps, and how much oxygen your muscles use when you're exercising vigorously are the best measure of your overall fitness. This measure is called your "maximum breathing capacity." It's your aerobic power.

Walking briskly. Running. Cross-country skiing. Jumping rope. Using aerobic machines such as a stationary bike, treadmill, or rowing machine. Vigorous, nonstop studio exercises like those in my Workout. —All these are aerobic activities. They work like this: Sustained, rhythmic contractions of the large leg and hip muscles press against the blood vessels so that they send increased amounts of blood to the heart. This makes the heart work harder. The heart is a muscle and, like any muscle, becomes larger and stronger when worked—though only to a certain percentage of its capacity and for a limited length of time. As the heart muscle becomes stronger, it pumps more blood through the circulatory system with fewer beats. And since it's blood that carries oxygen through the body, when more blood is pumped, more oxygen is available to the muscles for the production of energy.

In addition to its positive effects on the heart, aerobic exercise multiplies the number of oxygen-carrying cells in your blood and improves the ability of the enzymes in your muscles to extract this oxygen. It increases the number of capillaries—the smallest blood vessels—that bring blood to the muscles. It also enlarges the arteries—the largest blood vessels. As a result, the blood pressure decreases. The blood's ability to dissolve harmful clots is improved. And levels of harmful fats in the blood are reduced while levels of healthful fat substances, HDLs, are increased. These are the high-density lipoproteins that speed harmful fats and cholesterol through the bloodstream before they can be deposited as plaque inside the blood vessels.

## HOW TO DO AEROBIC EXERCISES EFFECTIVELY:

- To be truly effective, aerobic exercise must be done *briskly*—raising the pulse rate to approximately *75 percent* of the maximum number of times your heart can beat in a minute. This is called your Training Heart Rate. This should be your training *goal*. To achieve it, be sure to begin your exercise program at a 60 percent training rate and build up gradually to your ideal 75 percent over a period of a month or two. Exercise below a 60 percent level will do much less to enhance your health or maintain your weight.
- Avoid exercising so hard and so fast that you are gasping for air. When you're out of breath, you are exercising *an*aerobically—without oxygen. The muscles are demanding oxygen faster than your cardiorespiratory system is able to deliver it. Without sufficient oxygen, the muscles will quickly fatigue. In addition, if we are exercising to lose or maintain our weight, our effort becomes counterproductive when it's anaerobic. That's because anaerobic exercise uses stored carbohydrates or glycogen as its only fuel. Aerobic exercise, on the other hand, mobilizes *fat* as its major fuel. And fat is only burned up in the presence of *lots of oxygen*.
- Aerobic exercise must be *steady and sustained* for at least 20 to 30 minutes —depending on the intensity of the aerobics you are doing. Theoretically you can continue for up to an hour if you want to.
- Aerobic exercise should be *regular and consistent*—at least three times a week to maintain your aerobic fitness and up to six times to improve it.
- Remember, from a calorie-burning point of view, it is better to continue an activity for a longer time at a more moderate pace than to do it harder for a shorter time. If, for instance, a 150-pound runner jogged one mile in 12 minutes, she (or he) would burn 110 calories. This slow pace would

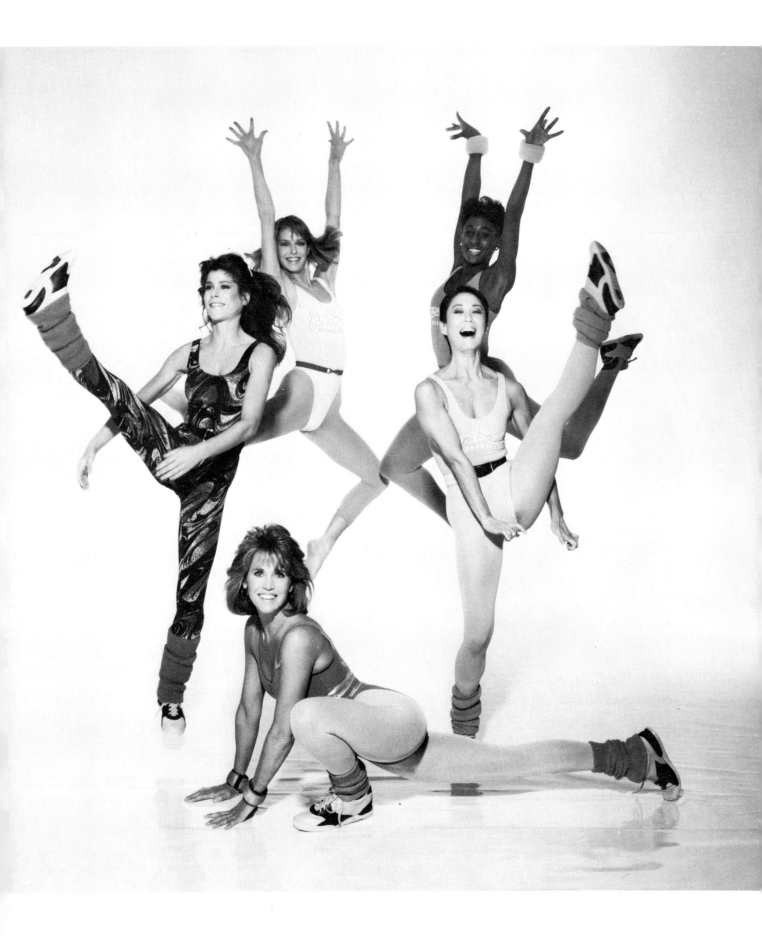

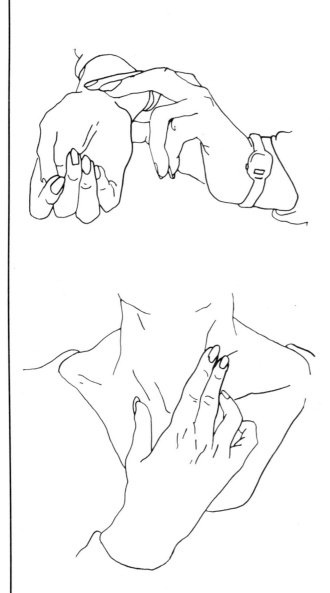

## THE PULSE:
## YOUR COACH WITHIN

Here's how you can use your pulse to determine if your workout is aerobically effective.

### Find Your Training Rate:

Your target training range is 60–85 percent of your maximum heart rate. The ideal training goal is 75 percent.

**(Be sure to begin at the lower end of your target range and build up slowly.)**

To find your maximum heart rate, subtract your age from 220 beats a minute, which is everyone's maximum heart rate in early adulthood. This number is your maximum heart rate.

Now multiply this number by 60 percent, 75 percent, and then 85 percent to find the lower, middle, and upper ranges of intensity for your aerobic exercise.

### Check Your Training Rate:

Immediately after exercising, take your pulse for 10 seconds. Multiply this by 6 to calculate how many times your heart has been beating per minute during exercise. Use either the pulse in your wrist or the carotid artery in your neck. If you are a newcomer to exercise, this pulse rate should be approximately 60 percent of your maximum heart rate. If you are very fit it should be in the 85 percent range.

NOTE: A few high-blood-pressure medications lower the maximum heart rate and thus the training rate. If you're taking high-blood-pressure medication, call your physician to find out if your exercise program needs to be adjusted.

probably permit her to keep going. If she jogged three miles she would burn 330 calories. If this same person ran one mile in a very fast 5 minutes and 30 seconds she would burn about 130 calories, but she would probably not be able to continue running much longer, and chances are she would end up burning fewer calories than her slower fellow-joggers who could keep going longer.

# RUNNING

Running is an excellent form of aerobic exercise that costs nothing and can be done almost anywhere—on the high-school track, on a quiet suburban street, along a country road, on the beach, in the park, even around your house or driveway or the supermarket parking lot before the supermarket opens in the morning.

There was a time when I never dreamed I could jog or run. I had gone running a few times with men, but every time I did my chest would ache and I would be gasping for breath within minutes. I had also heard that running gave you big leg muscles, made your bottom drop, and was bad for a woman's reproductive organs. That settled it. Running was not for me.

Then several years later, I tried again. Three women friends who were regular runners invited me to go running with them one evening. They were going to run along the Pacific Palisades, a beautiful stretch that overlooks the ocean near where we live. I was surprised at how easy it was. We ran along chatting with each other and when we started to pant, we would stop and walk. I suddenly realized that I loved it. I felt great. And so proud of myself! I could do it! I realized that my mistake before was in trying to run too fast, competing with men who were experienced runners.

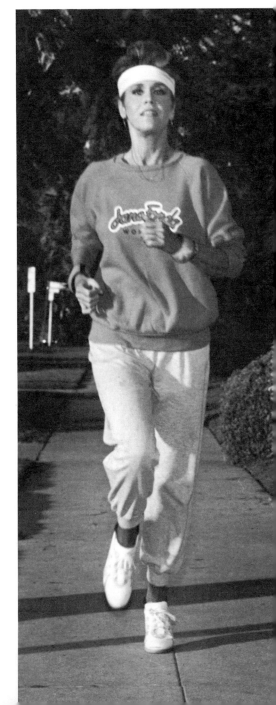

After this experience, I began to take running seriously. I would start very slowly and when I began to pant would drop down to a brisk walk for a while and then jog again. Little by little my jogging time grew longer and the walking time shorter. I was really excited when I jogged my first mile.

When I finally reached the two-mile mark, I got too cocky. The next day I abruptly increased my distance to three miles and began running three miles a day, every day, at a time when I was very tired. I paid for this mistake with a painful "runner's knee" and could not run for three weeks.

This started me reading books on running, something I encourage you to do before you start running yourself. I learned how important it is to increase your distance *gradually,* that you should not be compulsive about running the maximum distance every day, and that you should learn to listen to your body. If it tells you that you are tired, don't push too hard.

I am reminded of a poem by Lao Tzu whose wisdom I still try to keep in mind:

> For all things there is a time for going ahead and a time for following behind,
>> A time for slow breathing and a time for fast breathing,
>>> A time to grow in strength and a time to decay,
>>> A time to be up and a time to be down.
>> Therefore, the sage avoids all extremes, excesses, and extravagances.

As for all those dire forecasts that I used to believe about running—well, it may not be the ideal exercise for some people, because it does put stress on your knee and hip joints. And it may not be indicated for women with fragile reproductive organs. I am not qualified to say. I do know, however, that if you have the proper running shoes and come down on your heels first rather than your toes, you will not build large leg muscles nor will your bottom drop. On the contrary, the muscles in your buttocks, hips, thighs, and legs will be strengthened, and, judging from my own experience, if you keep your pulse rate up to your training level long enough, you will be

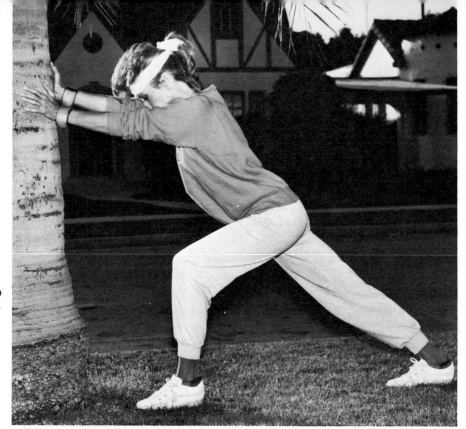

*It's important always to stretch before and after you run.*

shedding fat in those problem areas. And if you take a few minutes to warm up, and stretch before and after your run, your muscles will stay long and flexible and you'll have less risk of injury.

I love running now. I try to do six or seven miles several times a week and three or four miles on off-days. I have run through the dappled summer light of country roads in New England, chugged around indoor tracks so small that I felt like a hamster on an exercise wheel, run in Central Park in New York when it was so cold my tears froze, and dragged myself bleary-eyed into the California dawn to get my run in before the children woke up.

I love that it gets me outside and turns my skin pink all over. I enjoy seeing the familiar faces of fellow runners, particularly those feisty over-60s. I like that it is free, that you can do it anywhere, and I especially love it when it's over.

## WALKING

I have recently added walking and hiking to my exercise repertoire. They're the most natural forms of aerobic exercise. At our family's ranch, high in the hills north of Santa Barbara, I can get all the exercise I need in the most pleasurable of ways: climbing up and down beautiful wild hills, becoming familiar with the smells, rocks, flowers, and wildlife so unique to Southern California.

At the Workout Studios, our early morning "Walkout" classes have become increasingly popular as people discover the pleasures and effectiveness of walking. It places little pressure on the joints and lower back, so there's rarely a risk of injury. Its benefits match those of running—you just have to do it longer. Every mile walked, for instance, burns essentially the same number of calories as every mile run—about 110. Going farther and for a longer period of time, rather than speeding up, is what counts from an aerobic standpoint.

Walking any old way won't do, however, if it's fitness you're after. Here are a few basic tips:

- *Walk briskly*—four or five miles in an hour is a realistic goal.
- *Walk with weight slightly forward.* Push off from the back toes instead of grabbing with the front heel. The feet should point as straight ahead as possible and the legs should be aligned with your hips.
- *Take long, stretching strides,* working your legs and buttocks to their maximum.
- *Think tall,* chest lifted, back flat, and head up—erect but not rigid.
- *Swing your arms vigorously,* wide and free like a pendulum.
- *Walk relaxed.*

Eventually, if you want to increase the aerobic challenge of walking, you can add weights to your wrists or waist. (You can add as much as 20 percent of your body weight, but be sure to do so *gradually*.) I recommend the one-pound Spenco wrist weights that we use at the Workout. I *don't* recommend using ankle weights when you walk. They put too much stress on the knees and other joints.

To prevent injury from both walking *and* running, make a habit of doing five to ten minutes of slow stretching before you start and after you finish—especially afterward. Emphasize stretching the backs of the legs—the calves and the backs of the thighs or hamstrings. You'll find excellent calf and hamstring stretches on pages 107–109, 133, and 162–163 of the Workout exercises.

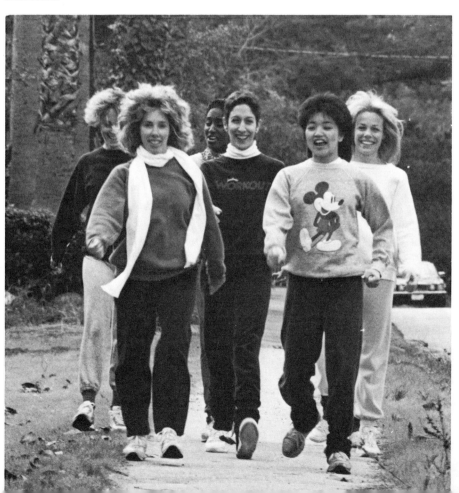

## MACHINES: PASSIVE RESISTANCE

It seems most of my new exercise experiences happen as a result of breaking my feet. One broken foot got me started with my Workout regime. Another time when I was in Israel I broke my foot late at night running to answer the telephone in a strange apartment. I turned the wrong way and fell downstairs. This happened only weeks before I had to begin filming *On Golden Pond,* where once more I had to wear a bikini—and do that back flip. I could not afford to wait until the cast came off to get into shape. There just wasn't time. I had to start almost immediately, cast be damned!

I went to classes at my Workout Studio and did what I could with that big plaster lump weighing me down. But it wasn't enough. In desperation I went to a gym equipped with Nautilus machines.

The whole notion of using machines and weights left me cold. They seemed absolutely contrary to my dancer's sensibilities. I soon learned, however, that many dancers use machines, and they are helpful for anyone with an injury. Working out on a series of machines is called circuit training. Each machine uses isolated muscle groups so you can quite safely work your body while avoiding the injured area.

There are different kinds of equipment—Nautilus, Universal, Camm II, Eagle, and others. You can get a good workout on all of them if you know how to use them. It really depends on which equipment is most convenient for you.

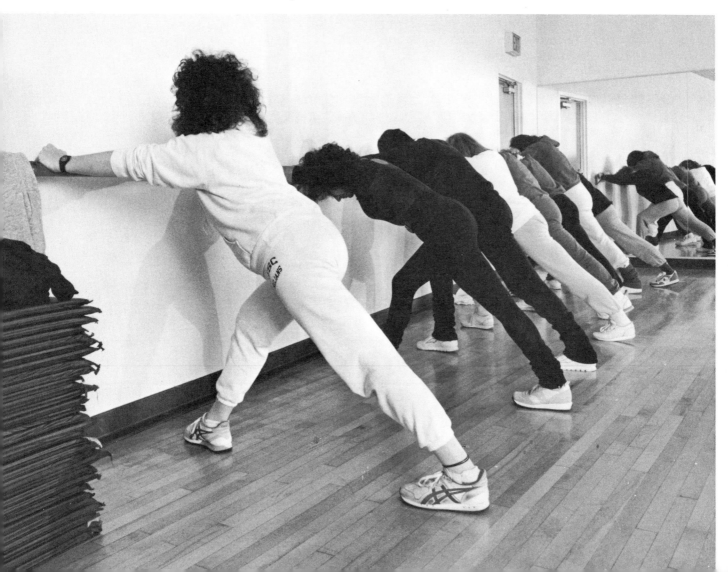

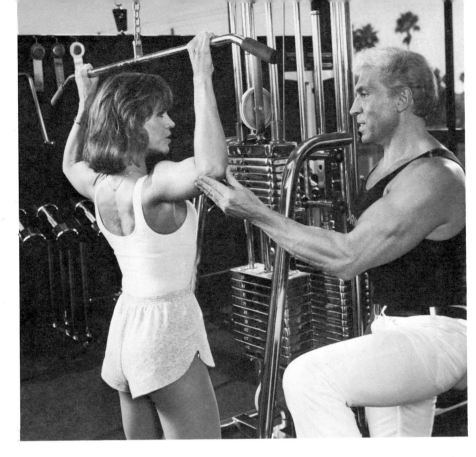

I am disturbed by how often I see people using equipment incorrectly, because they are not getting the most out of the time and energy they are spending. Ideally you should have a trainer with you when you use the machines. If the gym you go to does not provide individual training, try to find a trainer somewhere else who can spend time giving you thorough instructions before you go it alone.

## MY PERSONAL EXERCISE REGIME

The keystone of my exercise program is my own Workout, which gives me the stretching I need to keep my muscles and ligaments (which link one bone to another) long and flexible. The exercises are rhythmic and sustained, so they provide cardiovascular conditioning. My Workout also includes exercises that are done against resistance, either that of my own body or wrist and ankle weights, so that I develop muscle tone.

I like having a routine that I can learn by heart and follow each day. This way I can compete with myself, keep track of how many repetitions I can do, and see for myself to what extent my strength and endurance is increasing. Also, I do my Workout to music, which makes it more fun.

I try to do the Workout at least three or four times a week. I find I work harder when I'm in a class, but when I have to travel or go away on a film location I bring my Workout videos with me and find it's almost like being in class. I usually alternate between the New Workout, which is similar to the program in this book, and the Challenge Workout, depending on how I feel, and for a greater change, I'll use the Stretch and Tone Workout tape on

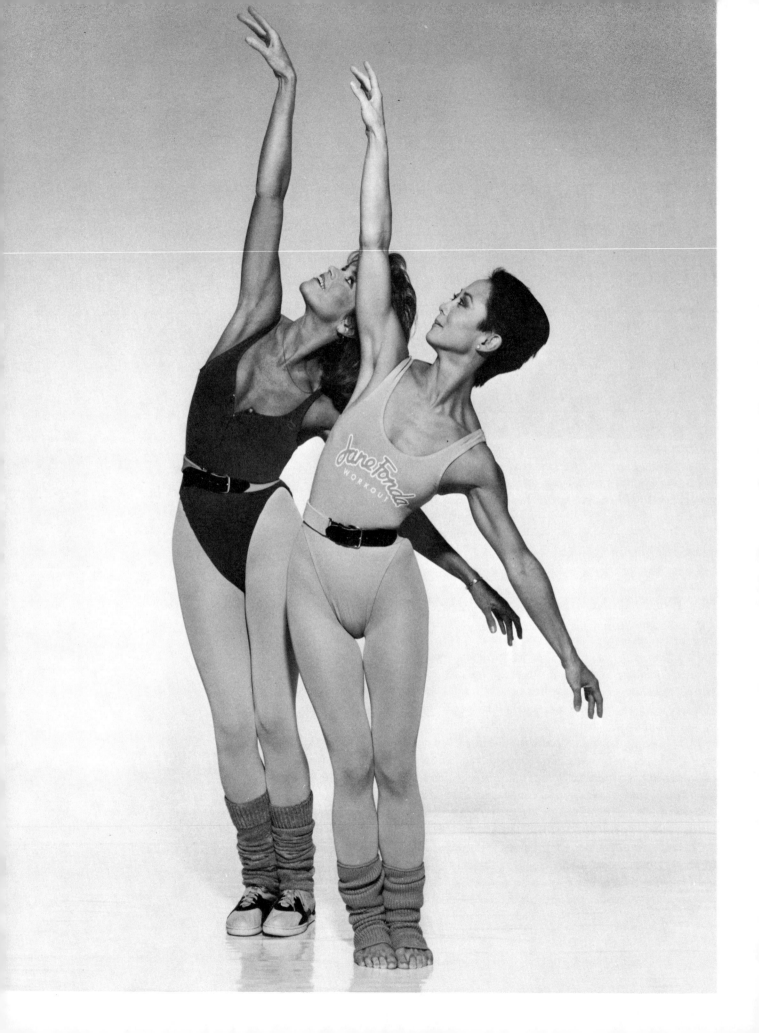

days when the idea of jumping up and down seems overwhelming. It's funny, but when I'm exercising to my own record or video I don't see myself as "Jane" but as that loudmouthed drill sergeant who's always promising "it's almost over" when it never seems to end. I find myself telling her to "shut up" a lot . . . but I do keep going.

When I'm preparing to do a film and want to get into super shape, I combine the Workout with circuit-training on weight machines and some upper body work with dumbbells (free weights). I try to do the Workout three or four times a week and weight-training two or three times a week. On the days when I do weight-training, which is not aerobic, I try to supplement it with at least 30 minutes of aerobics at my training level on a stationary bike, or rowing machine, or running or walking. I always rest at least once a week—and, let's be honest, there are plenty of times when my schedule prohibits exercise altogether. Occasionally, a week will go by when I simply don't have time to do anything but stretch. At those times, I really feel the difference in my energy level and sense of overall wellness.

Incidentally, if you have gone off your exercise routine for a week or more, don't try to jump right back in at the same level. Your muscles will have lost some of their ability to use oxygen efficiently. No matter how fit you are, it takes only three to four weeks to become unconditioned. So if you have to stop exercising for one reason or another, don't feel bad that you cannot exercise at your previous level. Don't even try. Give your body a chance to rev up again.

## WORKOUT CLASS

When you are checking out an exercise class, here are seven things to look for:

1. There should be a warm-up at the beginning of class. Warming up includes stretching and getting your pulse rate up. This helps your metabolic system get itself ready for the exercises that follow. The blood vessels in your muscles will expand and be prepared for receiving an increased flow of blood. The harder you work out—whether by jogging or some other form of aerobics, using machines, or following a program of calisthenics—the more you should stretch, since heavily worked muscles tend to become shorter and more easily pulled.

2. There should be a cool-down at the end of class. Cooling down at the end of vigorous exercise is extremely important. While you exercise, an increased amount of blood is pumped to your heart with the help of contractions in the large leg muscles that press against the veins. If your leg muscles relax abruptly, the blood will collect in your extremities (athletes refer to this as "pooling") instead of getting back to your heart. Your heart is still pumping hard, but no blood is going up. When you slow down gradually, your muscles continue to assist in pumping up the blood until your pulse rate subsides, less blood is being pumped, and your heart can handle it on its own.

   During the cool-down, the muscles also are able to expel the toxic wastes produced by the metabolic process more easily.

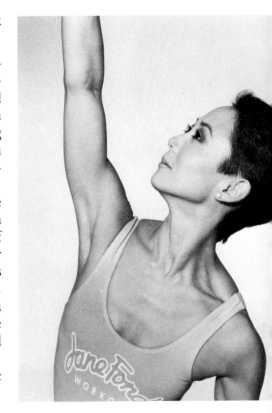

3. The instructor's movements should be clear and precise so that you can follow them easily.
4. The instructor should demonstrate an understanding of the body and be concerned that students are doing each exercise correctly. You should be able to tell that she or he enjoys teaching and works to motivate each student to extend herself to her limits.
5. The exercise routine should be challenging, but beware of teachers who believe that faster and harder is better than longer and more moderate. You'll risk injury and not be working aerobically if you aren't careful.
6. The surface upon which you are working out should provide enough spring to minimize undue stress to the shins, joints, and lower back. Carpet or padding over concrete floors is to be avoided.
7. When class is over, you should find yourself standing straighter and feeling exhilarated.

## DEBUNKING A FEW EXERCISE MYTHS

- Don't wear a vinyl or rubber garment while exercising. Because it prevents evaporation of sweat—our natural cooling system—the vinyl forces the body's temperature up at a time when fluid reserves are down. This can result in dangerous dehydration and overheating.
- There is no reason to stop exercising during menstruation. In fact, exercise has been shown to help relieve menstrual cramps in many women.
- Muscle does *not* turn into fat. Unused muscle can weaken, shrink in size, and be *replaced* by fat, but muscles don't become fat.
- Some people who are trying to lose weight avoid exercise because they think it will increase their appetite. Not true. Rigorous (but not excessive) exercise depresses appetite.
- And finally, the question of spot reducing: There is no basis to the claim that exercising one part of the body will reduce the fat in that area. Exercise mobilizes fat from stores *throughout* the body, not from an isolated area that is being exercised. However, repetitive exercise using an isolated group of muscles does build and tone those muscles, giving an esthetic result as well as raising basal metabolism.

Please remember that your goal is not to get pencil-thin or to look like someone else. Your goal should be to take your body and make it as healthy, strong, flexible, and well-proportioned as you can. Thin or plump, young or old, you will be more beautiful and have a prouder carriage, healthier glow, and a supple flow of movement which says that you are comfortable and confident about your physical self.

A wonderful by-product of all these activities is that you will find new interests beginning to open up in your life.

Like me, you may never have thought of yourself as an athletic, outdoorsy sort of person. You were an observer. Sitting it out. Always a little too tired or worried that you wouldn't perform well enough. Group sports, camping trips, exploring one of our magnificent national parks were for other folks, probably of Scandinavian descent.

Since I started running and exercising regularly, I have developed a real desire to do these things. I need to be outside more. I seek clean air and natural beauty, and I'm always open to new activities because I have the stamina to do them. I don't want to be a bystander anymore. I want to participate, not necessarily to achieve excellence, but just to have fun.

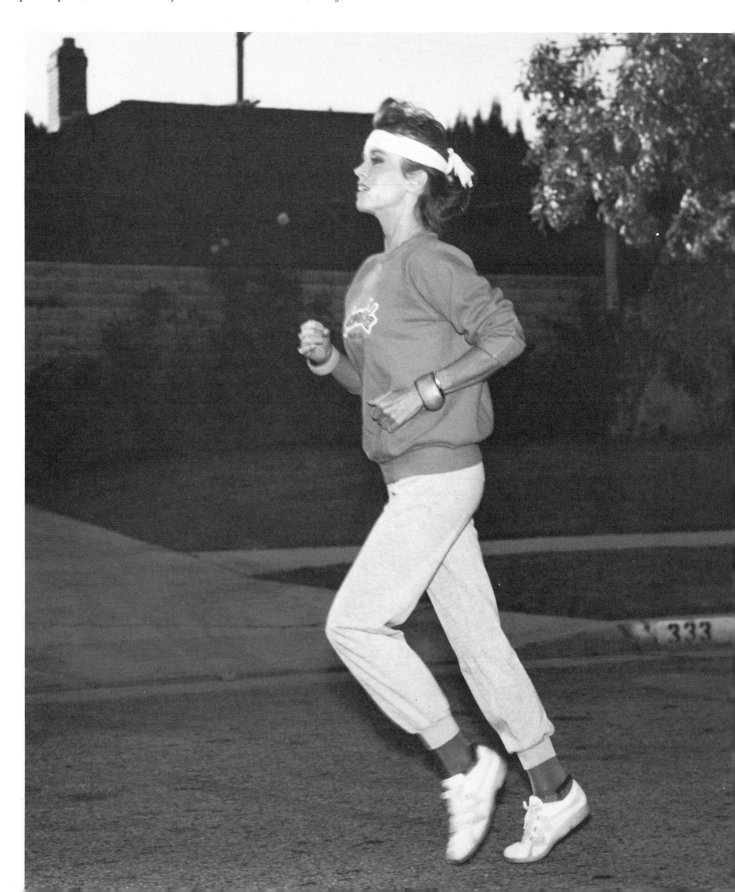

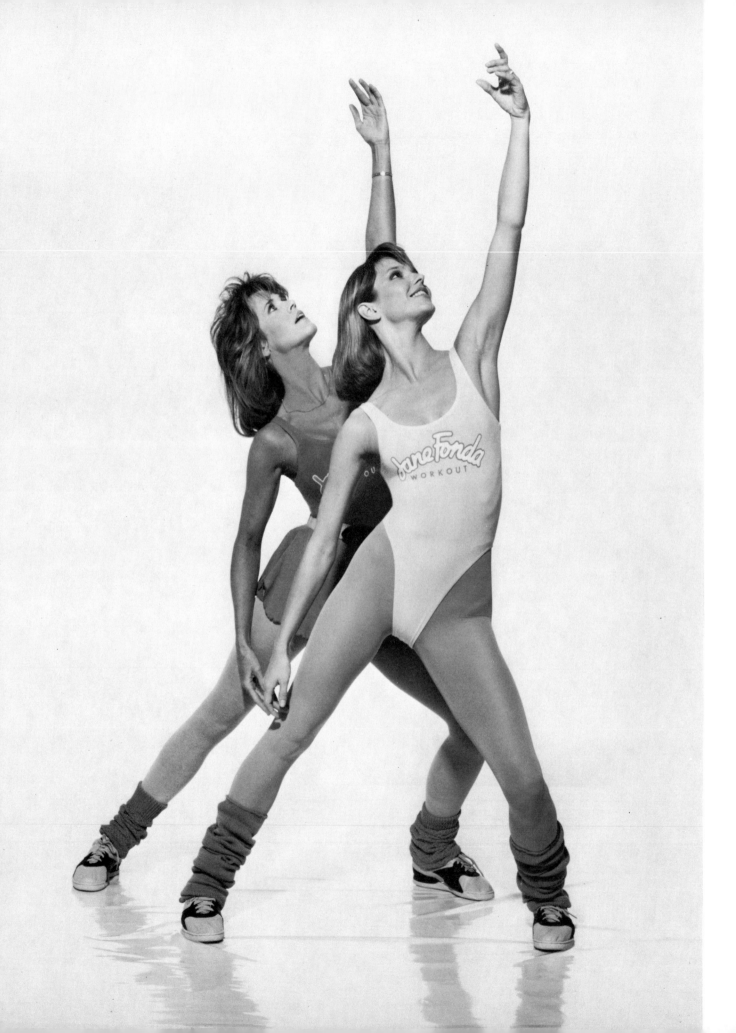

# UNDERSTANDING THE NEW WORKOUT

I never imagined years ago when I wrote my first book and produced my first record and videotape that doing the Workout would come to be called "doing Jane." I remember being on a plane the first time I heard this expression. A flight attendant came up to me and said "I want to thank you. My roommate and I 'do Jane' every day and I've never felt better." I've heard countless versions of this since. Sometimes it's a husband who laughingly says, "My wife does you every morning. Boy, am I sick of your voice!" Or sometimes it's a mother who tells me about losing twenty pounds "doing Jane" with her little girl.

It's very gratifying to me that "doing Jane" has had such a positive effect on so many people's lives. And as I had hoped, the results reported back to me person-to-person or in letters demonstrate not only weight loss, but also reduced stress, increased energy, more interest in nutrition, more motivation to become involved in sports, less need for medication, and many other life-enhancing benefits.

Now I have developed a New Workout. This is the basic exercise program we now teach at my Workout Studios and which I myself do regularly. (It's available on record and videotape as well.) I have revised the original Workout because a great deal more has been learned about exercise physiology and the science of aerobics in the four years that have elapsed since I wrote my first book. The New Workout represents everything I've discovered during that time. It's "state of the art," if you will. While for the most part there is no *one* way to exercise each particular part of the body, the New Workout incorporates the latest knowledge about the best and most effective ways to work different muscle groups.

Its exercises are carefully structured to use each part of the body in a specific sequence. You may be tempted to go straight to the ones that attack your trouble spots, and skip the other exercises. This is all right once in a while when you're short of time. But on a regular basis you'd be missing the essence of the Workout. In order to have a real impact on your level of fitness, to burn up your stores of fat, to tone and strengthen your muscles, and to develop cardiovascular endurance, you must use your entire body in vigorous and sustained exercise for at least 30 minutes a session. This means putting yourself through the thorough paces of the whole Workout.

Together with its aerobic component, the basis of the New Workout is the repetition of certain movements that use a single muscle group against the resistance of your own body weight. We work each muscle group to its

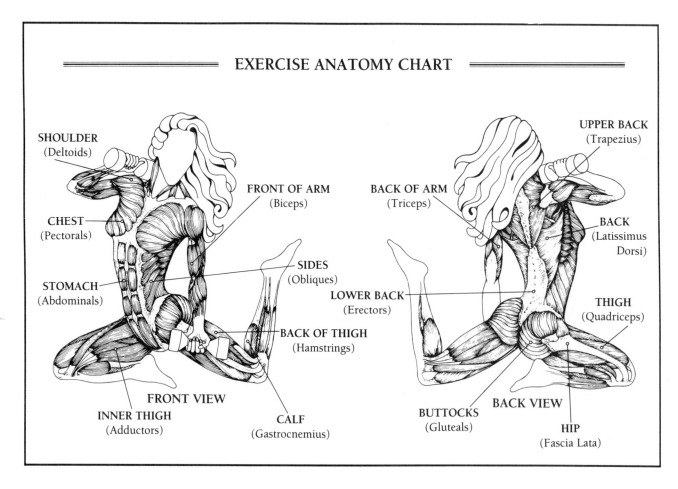

## EXERCISE ANATOMY CHART

**SHOULDER** (Deltoids)

**CHEST** (Pectorals)

**STOMACH** (Abdominals)

**FRONT OF ARM** (Biceps)

**SIDES** (Obliques)

**BACK OF THIGH** (Hamstrings)

**INNER THIGH** (Adductors)

**FRONT VIEW**

**CALF** (Gastrocnemius)

**UPPER BACK** (Trapezius)

**BACK OF ARM** (Triceps)

**BACK** (Latissimus Dorsi)

**LOWER BACK** (Erectors)

**THIGH** (Quadriceps)

**BACK VIEW**

**BUTTOCKS** (Gluteals)

**HIP** (Fascia Lata)

maximum. The repetitions are followed by stretches to develop flexibility and to keep your muscles long. The stretches are every bit as important as the repetitions.

If you are prepared to commit yourself to regular exercise, there is no question that you will alter the shape of your body, burn away those fatty deposits, and develop muscle tone where you never knew you could have it.

## WEIGHTS

For most of you the weight of your body will provide sufficient resistance during the repetitions, but by the time you have worked up to the advanced exercises, or if you are already accustomed to exercise, you may find that your muscles have grown used to your body weight. If you can get through the advanced Workout fairly easily without feeling undue discomfort, then instead of increasing the number of repetitions, you may want to add ankle or wrist weights.

A muscle is composed of fibers—the larger the muscle, the more fibers it contains. To get the full use of your muscles, all the fibers should be called into action. But your muscles will use only the number of fibers that they really need. At first it will take all the fibers in your abdominal muscles to lift your legs up when you are on your back, but when these muscles get stronger they will only need to use a fraction of their fibers. And that is all they will use no matter how many leg lifts you do. This means it is time to add weights.

My advanced students at the Workout use snug, half-pound to one-pound weights on their wrists during the upper body exercises. This is more advisable than holding weights in your hands. You want to have your hands free and flexible during upper body work. For the abdominal and leg work my students use as much as two and a half to three pounds on their ankles (you can begin using just *half*-pound wrist and ankle weights and build up gradually). According to a study done by the Center for Sports and Dance Medicine at the St. Francis Hospital in San Francisco, one-pound wrist weights worn during the aerobic portion of the Workout will increase your aerobic output by 8 percent if you are very fit and by 12 percent if you are not very fit. We recommend the Spenco one-pound wrist weights. They are snug, which is important, and very pleasant to wear. Weights are available at all sporting goods stores.

You will not be able to do all the repetitions at first when you are wearing weights. That is all right. Do as many as you can before your muscles give out, and then go on to the next exercise. It is better to use all of a muscle for a short time than to do a hundred repetitions using only part of it.

If you are worried about developing bulging muscles, don't be. Women— 99.9 percent of us—do not have enough testosterone, the male hormone that governs muscle growth, to develop bulgy muscles. But something does happen to your muscles, and I like it. Since you are reading this book, you are probably like me and appreciate a woman's body on which the muscle cuts and contours are evident. This is what you will get with regular workouts.

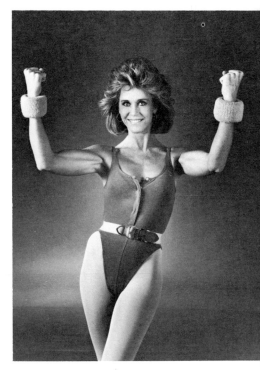

*At the Workout we use these 1-pound Spenco wrist weights.*

## PREPARING FOR YOUR WORKOUT

1. Try to set a regular time to exercise. I prefer working out early in the morning. I get it out of the way and start the day with high energy. You may find it easier to do after work, if you've been sitting all day and the tension has built up. Or the afternoon, when the baby is sleeping, may be the best for you.

   Exercise in the early evening can relax you, relieve tension, and help keep you from overeating at dinner. In the afternoon it can serve as a pick-me-up and revitalize you for the rest of the day. Choose the time that suits your schedule best and then stick to it. Getting a routine going is half the battle. But don't feel you have failed if you miss a workout for some good reason. The guilt will make you feel discouraged and that old self-punishment syndrome—eating—might set in.

2. Turn the phone off before you start.

3. You need a place to exercise where there is no draft and the ceiling is high enough to allow you to jump up and clap your hands overhead. You need room enough to swing your arms wide without hitting anything.

4. You need an exercise pad or towel or blanket to give you a little padding

for your floor work. If you are on a carpet, put a towel down to delineate your workout space and keep the dust fibers out of your nose and hair.

5. Dress for it. An exercise outfit helps because it sets this time apart from the rest of your day and makes it matter more. I prefer a leotard and tights. If I'm feeling overweight, I put on a pair of those baggy sweatpants that feel like parachute silk with an elastic belt. They cover up a multitude of sins and help heat your body faster. I always wear leg warmers to keep my leg muscles warm—and because they make me feel like a dancer. You should feel comfortable and be able to move freely.

6. A big mirror to exercise in front of makes it a lot easier. Count yourself lucky if you have one. If not, it is not an essential.

7. Always make sure you are hydrated. This means drinking water a little before and also after exercise. Your goal should be eight glasses of water a day. Dehydration can dramatically reduce your energy and your exercise performance.

## MUSIC

My experience has been that exercising with music is easier and more fun. It helps motivate you and carries you along with more ease. I cannot even conceive of doing my workout without music.

Try to use music with the right rhythm, a steady easy-to-follow beat, and with a long enough running time so you won't have to get up and start it over more than once. Experiment a little. Make the music an important part of your routine.

I have produced a best-selling album as well as an audio cassette called "Jane Fonda's New Workout" on the CBS record label. It offers beginning and advanced exercises very similar to those in this book. I call out the instructions and count the repetitions accompanied by upbeat, motivating music. When I travel and carrying records is tough, I just bring my tape, a small tape recorder, and I'm all set.*

## HOW TO DO IT

In the beginning, it will seem very mechanical. You'll be trying to read the instructions and figure out when to breathe while trying all these new positions. Don't rush it. Read the instructions carefully. It is important that you do the exercises correctly, otherwise you risk getting hurt. And you won't be getting as much as you should from your efforts.

Memorize the exercise series as quickly as possible and then put the book away. The exercises are designed to flow from one to the next without

---

* You'll find how to obtain this album or cassette in the Workout Resources listings in the back of the book.

stopping, which is hard to do when you are following a book. So read and reread each section several times and go through the motions slowly to become familiar with them before you start with the music. It takes more time at the beginning, but it is worth it for the enjoyment you will have in moving from one section to the next.

Once you have reached this point, here is what you should do to have the most fun and get the most out of your workout.

1. Turn on the music you have chosen for the section, get in the correct starting position and—begin!
2. Go from one exercise to the next, and on and on without stopping until you have finished that section.
3. Stop.
4. Change the music and go on to the next section.
5. Do the exercises in the order indicated. They are designed to be done in sequence, one after the other. If no starting position is given, it means that the exercise begins in the same position where the one before it ended.
6. Maintain the momentum. This is extremely important. If you stop to answer the phone or whatever, your muscles will cool down. Cold muscles tear and sustain injury more easily. The cardiovascular benefits are lessened if your effort is not sustained. And psychologically, it is harder to start up again once you stop.

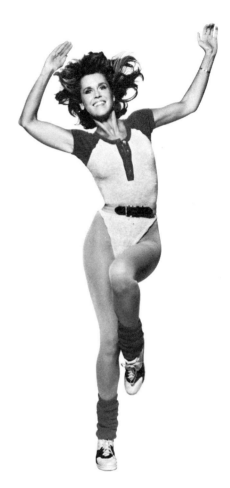

## BEGINNER OR ADVANCED?

You should start with the beginner's class unless you have had considerable exercise experience. Once you can do the beginner's workout all the way through smoothly and without strain, move up to the advanced class and gradually increase the number of repetitions to the amount indicated. Once you can do all the repetitions without strain, add the weights.

Do what you can. Don't push yourself too hard or you may get hurt. On the other hand, if it is easy it's not going to be effective. You have to challenge your body. Make yourself sweat. You always have to push a little beyond what you think you can do. You will be surprised at the untapped reserves of energy and strength you did not know you had.

When you think you can't do any more repetitions, do two more! Go for it!

## BREATHING

It is important to inhale and exhale as indicated. You may find that you have a tendency to hold your breath. Don't. You need to get that oxygen into your bloodstream. And you need to breathe out to eliminate waste products and toxic gases. In general, you should breathe out when you are making the most effort and breathe in when you ease up.

## TIPS

1. Newcomers to exercise may experience—as I did—muscle swelling. You will be looking forward to a looser fit in your slacks and to your horror you find they are tighter. Not to worry. You are working your muscles hard. It is as if someone punched them. They swell, but the swelling goes down very rapidly.
2. Pay more attention to losing inches than to losing pounds. Muscle weighs more than fat, so as you build strength your weight may stay the same or even increase slightly. But you will lose inches and your proportions will change for the better. To lose weight, you must cut back on your calories.
3. You will be stiff at first. You can minimize this by hopping into a hot bath after your workout before your muscles have cooled down. But do your exercises even if you are stiff. This will help dissipate the stiffness, and you will be surprised how quickly your muscles adapt as you maintain your routine. After the first week or so, you will probably not feel stiff any more.
4. Never eat within an hour before exercising. Your blood will be diverted to carry oxygen to your muscles just when it's needed to help in the digestive process, and this can nauseate you.
5. Always remember to empty your bladder before starting.

**One more thing . . .**

Just going through the motions won't get you the desired results. Concentrate on what you are doing. Concentrate on making your muscles work. Keep thinking about your posture and doing the exercises correctly.

**And finally . . .**

It takes work and time. You are about to begin something that I hope will become a permanent and pleasurable part of your life. Like most important endeavors, it will give back to you only what you put into it. Toning and firming can begin to show within days, but for a deep, total, and lasting effect, you need to work hard and regularly. If you do, you will find as I have that the rewards are immeasurable.

**It's time to get started.**

*opposite: Holding me up, as usual, are Julie LaFond, who runs the Workout (second from left), and Workout teachers who demonstrate the exercises in this book (l to r) Leslie Lilien, Angela Rodgers, Brigitte Steinberg, and Diane Toyama Ekker.*

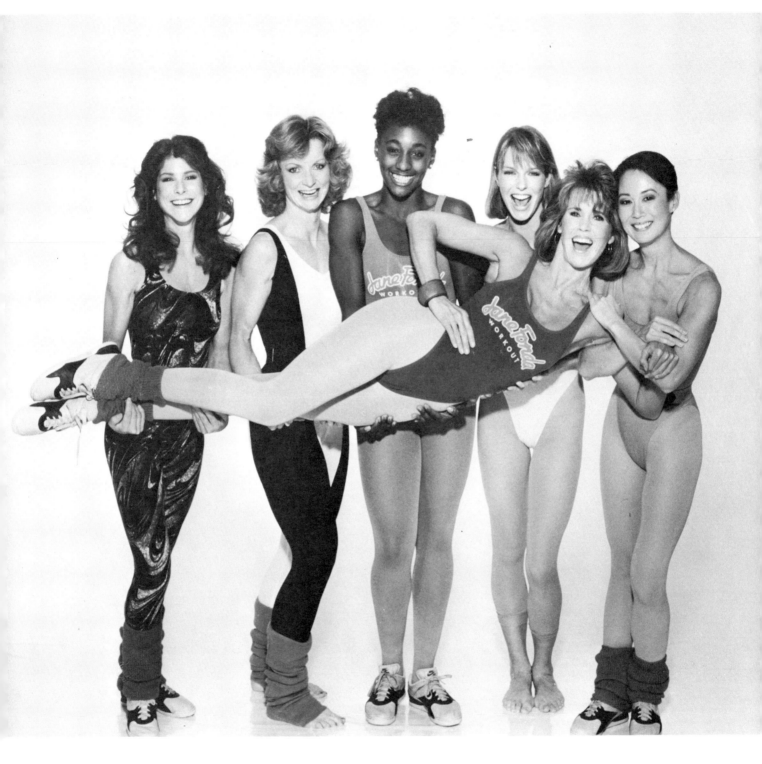

# III · THE NEW WORKOUT

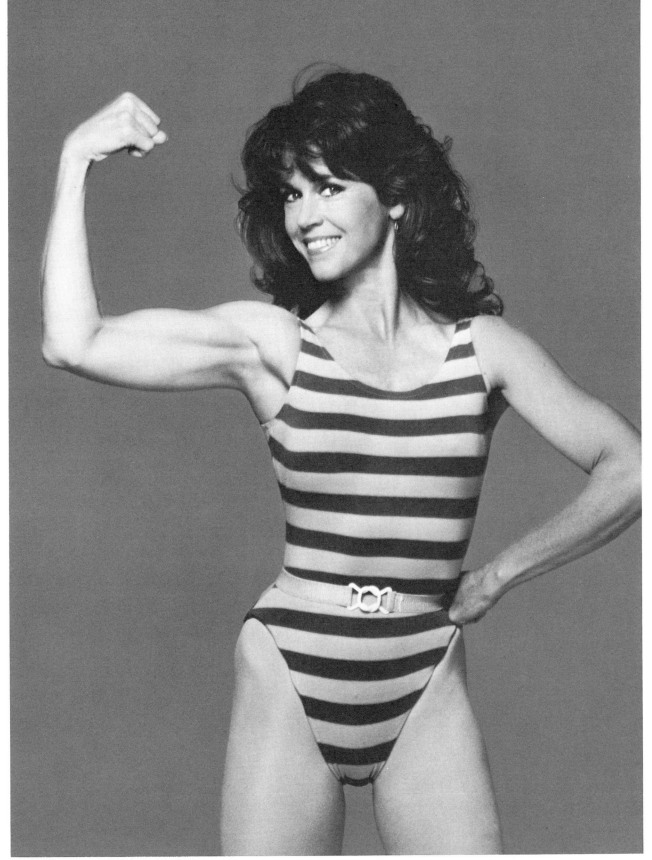

# BEGINNER'S WORKOUT

*Move smoothly in time to the music from one exercise to the next. Concentrate on doing the movements correctly, and making the muscles work deeply. Don't just go through the motions.*

**Correct Standing Posture:**

*Curl your pubic bone up toward your navel. Stomach should be pulled in, chest is lifted, shoulders are pressed back and down. Weight is slightly forward.*

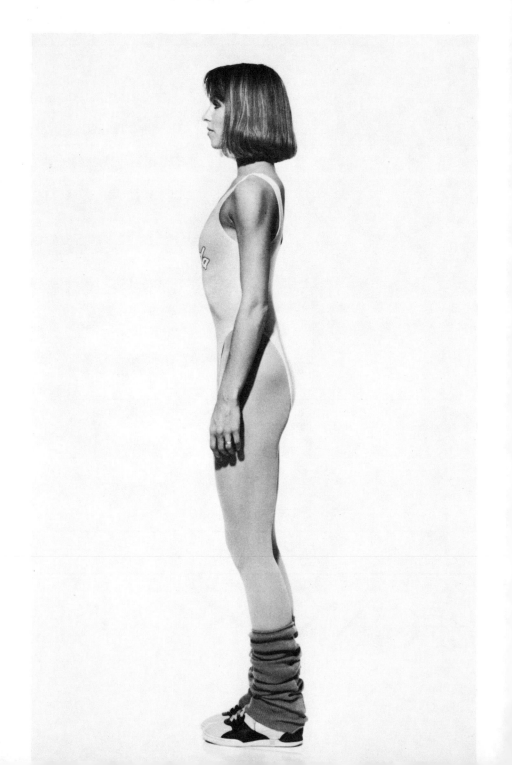

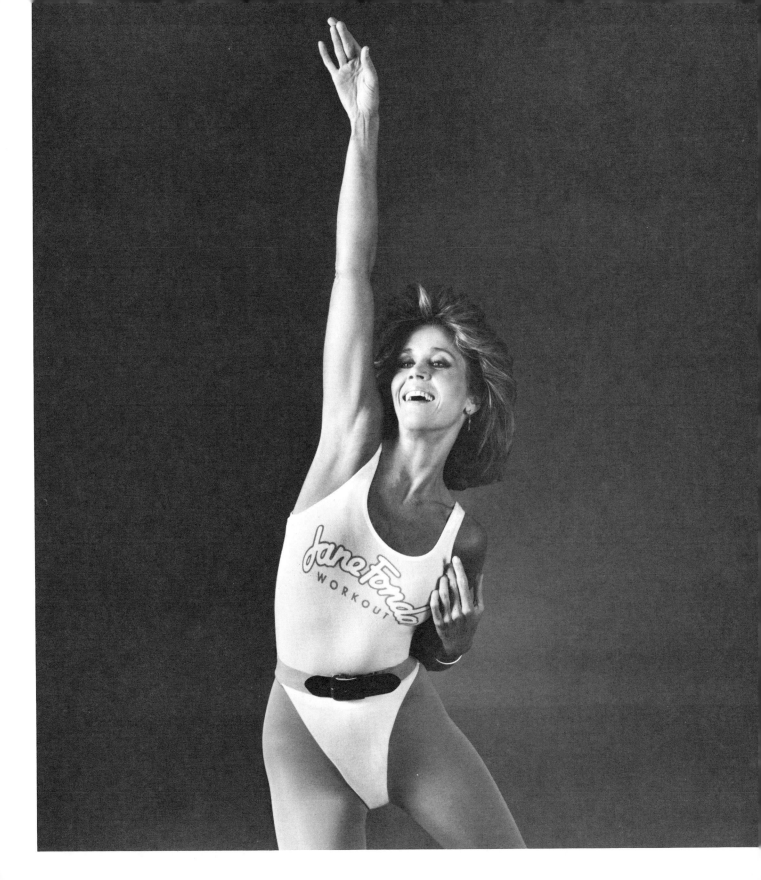

# Warm-up

*Starting position: Pull up tall from the waist, buttocks squeezed tight, stomach in, feet parallel a little more than hip-distance apart, knees slightly bent. Shoulders are pressed back and down.*

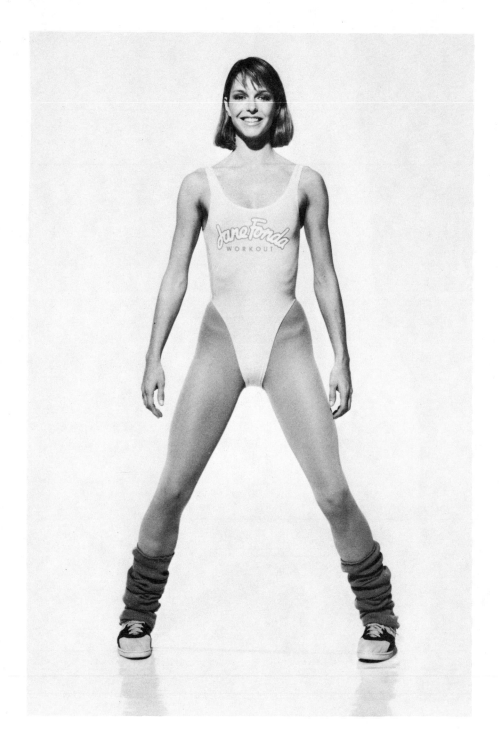

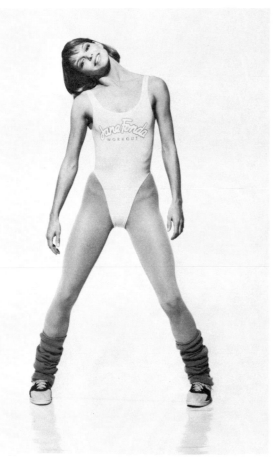

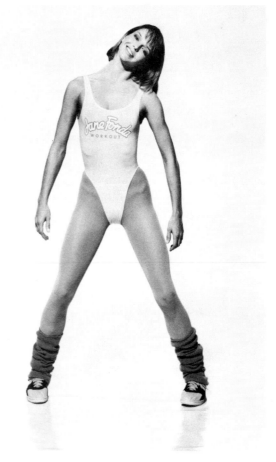

# 1 · HEAD PRESSES

1. Press your right ear toward your right shoulder and stretch for 4 counts. Feel the stretch in the left side of your neck. Be sure your shoulders are pressed back and down.

2. Press your left ear toward your left shoulder and stretch for 4 counts.

Repeat 4 counts to the right, 4 counts to the left.

3. Bring your head back to center.

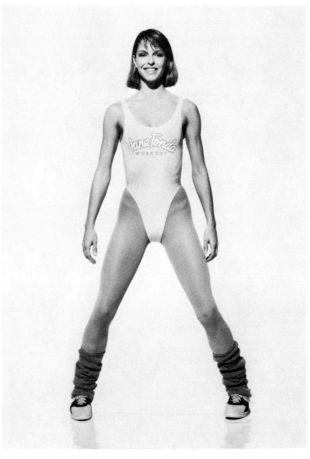

# 2 · SHOULDER ROLLS

1. Lift your shoulders up toward your ears, then circle them backward . . .

2. and down again in a big circle. Do 8 slow circles.

Be sure to get full motion in your shoulders and to keep your stomach pulled in, pubic bone tucked up, and weight slightly forward. Knees are still bent.

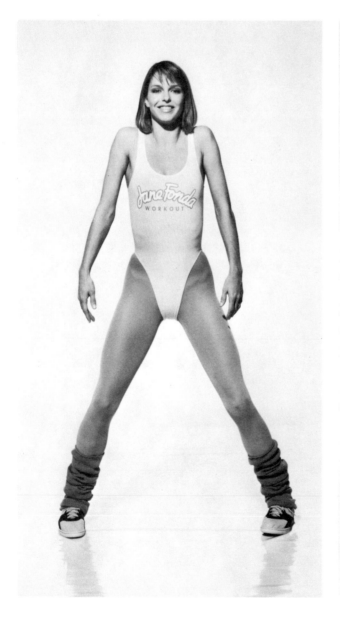 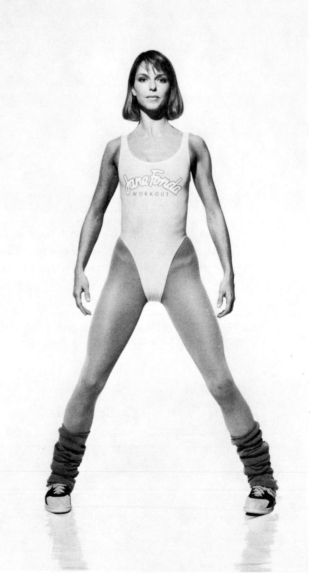

# 3 · ELBOW CIRCLES

1. Keep knees slightly bent. Place your hands on your shoulders, lift your elbows to the side at shoulder height, and circle your elbows forward and up . . .

2. then down and back 16 times.

Think of pressing your shoulder blades together as your elbows circle backward.

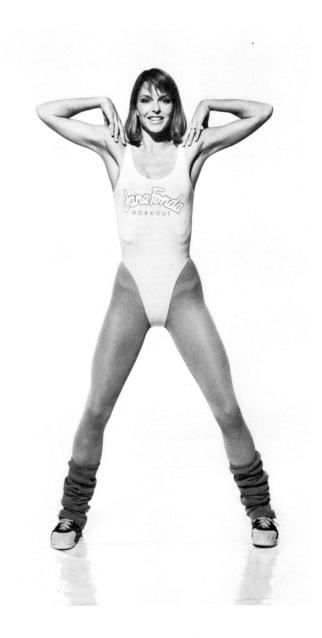
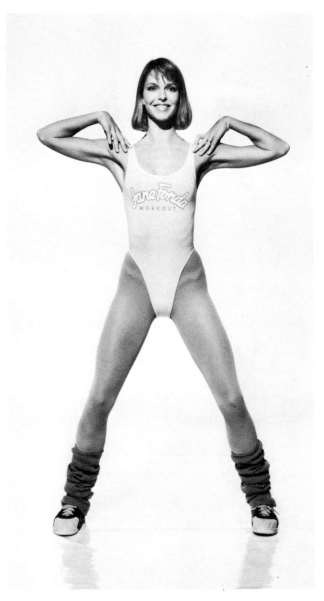

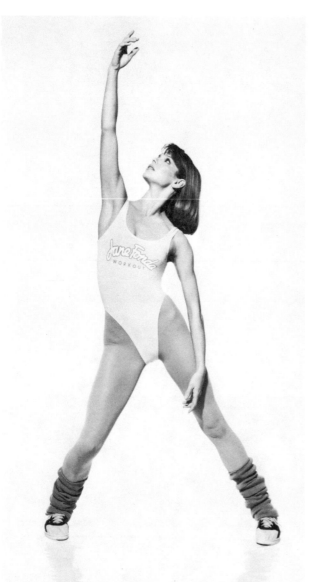 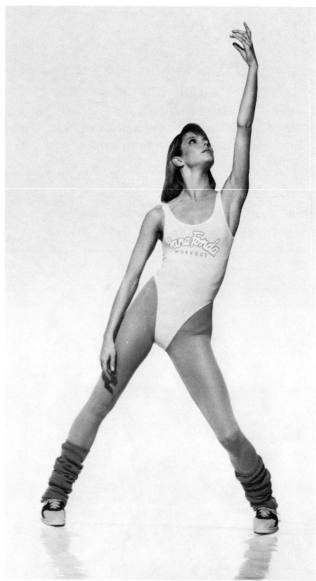

# 4 · WAIST LIFTS

1. With feet parallel, stretch your right arm upward as you bend your right knee. Feel a stretch up your right side.

2. Stretch your left arm upward as you bend your left knee. Feel a stretch up your left side.

Stretching right and left is 1 set. Repeat for a total of 8 sets.

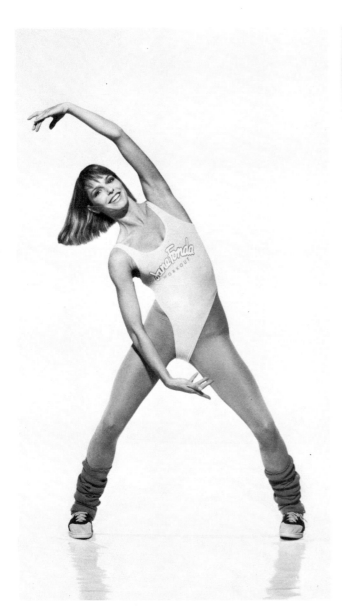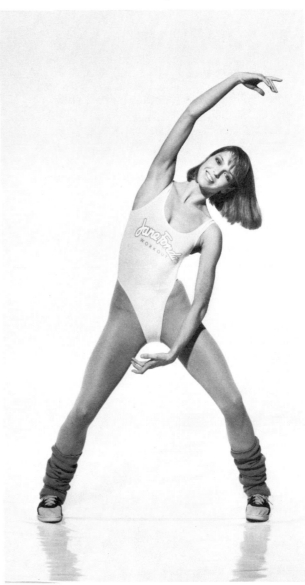

# 5 · WAIST REACHES

1. With feet still parallel and knees slightly bent, pull over to the right, reaching with your left arm over your head to the right, left shoulder pressed back, right arm curved in front of you. Stretch for 8 counts.

Don't let your left shoulder pull forward. Feel the stretch up your left side.

2. Reach over to the left side, stretching your right arm over your head to the left for 8 counts.

Don't let your right shoulder pull forward.

# 6 · SHOULDER STRETCH

1. Lace your fingers together behind your back. With knees bent, lean over and allow your arms to stretch forward over your head. Hold for 8 counts.

Your head should be relaxed, your back rounded.

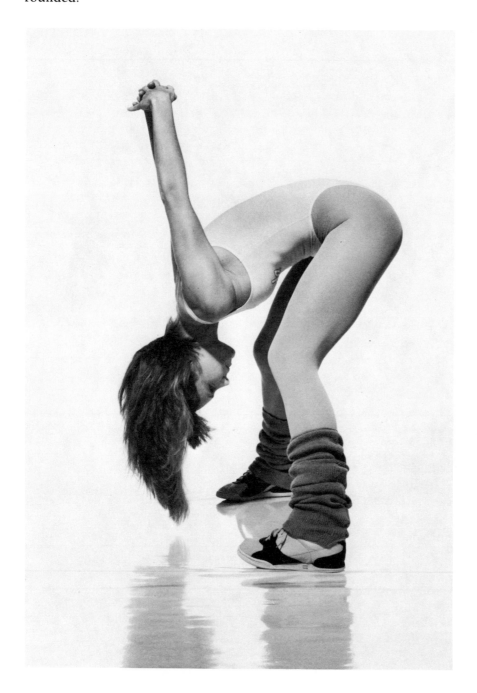

# 7 · HAMSTRING STRETCH

1. Knees slightly bent, clasp both ankles or calves. Stretch for 8 counts.

2. Slowly straighten your knees and gently press your chest toward your thighs. Stretch for 8 counts.

BREATHE DEEPLY.

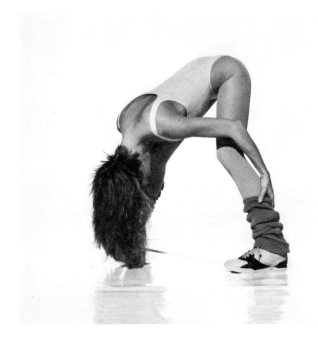

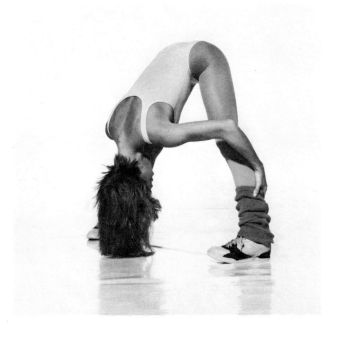

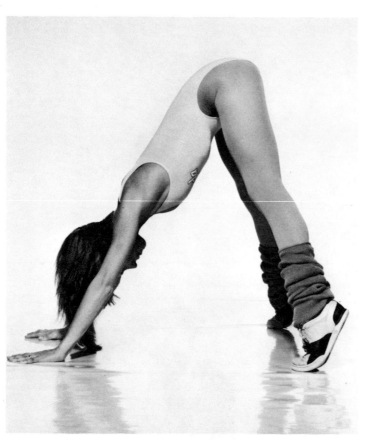

# 8 · TOE RAISES

1. Walk your hands out in front of you. With feet parallel press up very high on your toes . . .

2. then lower your heels. Press up and lower 20 times.

Keep your abdominals pulled in.

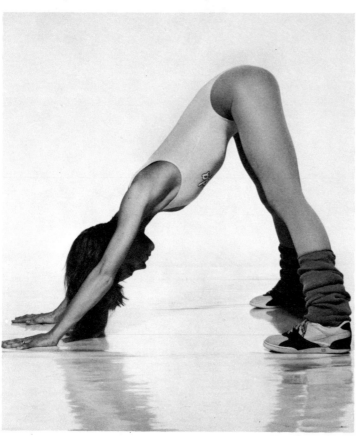

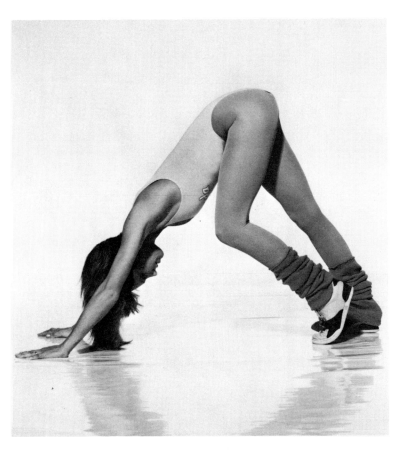

# $9 \cdot$ TENDON STRETCH

1. Walk your feet together to about 4 inches apart. Lift your left heel and bend your left knee as you press your right heel to the floor for 4 counts.

2. Lift your right heel, bending the right knee, as you press your left heel to the floor. Hold for 4 counts.

Right and left heel stretch is 1 set. Do 3 sets. Then press both heels toward the floor and hold for 4 counts.

Keep your abdominals pulled in. Feel the stretch up the back of the legs.

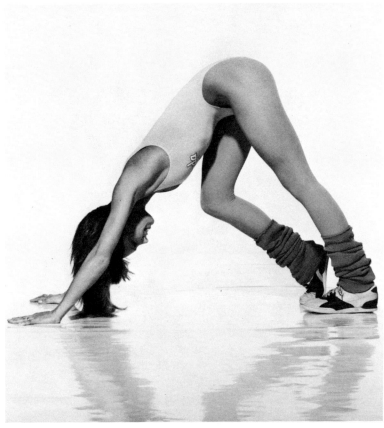

# 10 · KNEE BENDS

1. Walk your feet up to your hands. Place your hands on your lower legs and bend your right knee . . .

2. then your left knee.

Bending right and left is 1 set. Do 4 sets.

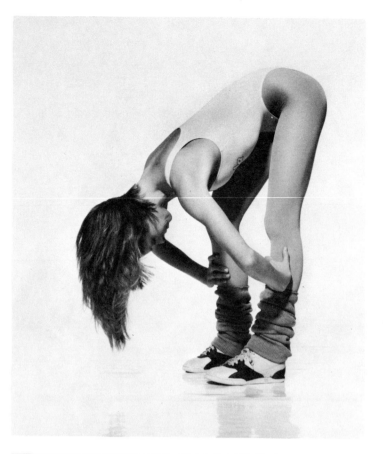

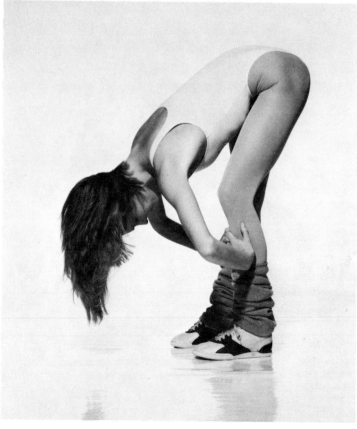

# 11 · PUSH-UPS

1. Get down on your hands and knees with your ankles crossed, feet high off the floor, and your hips pressing forward. Your back is flat. Weight is forward on your straight arms. Hands are beneath your shoulders pointing front.

Abdominals are pulled in. Buttocks are squeezed tight. *Do not arch your back.*

2. Inhale and bend your elbows, lowering your body as far as you can. Then exhale and straighten your arms again.

Do as many as you can without feeling strain in your lower back. One push-up may be all you can do at first. Build up gradually.

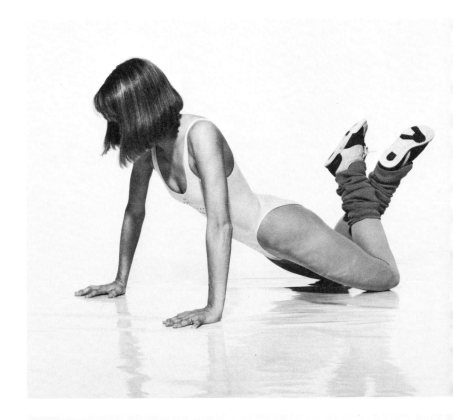

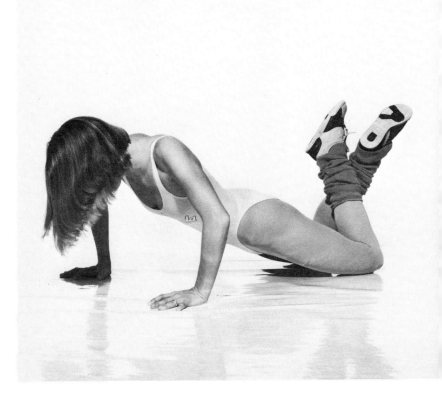

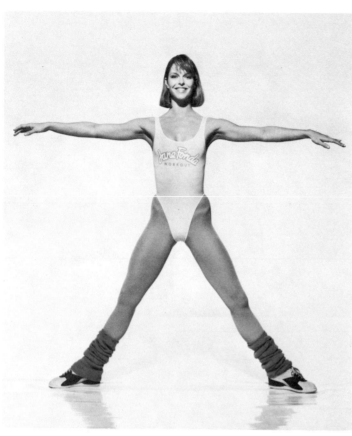

# 12 · PLIÉS

1. Stand with your legs *very* wide apart, feet *slightly* turned out, arms to the side at shoulder height.

2. Bend your knees so that your hips are almost on a level with your knees. Keep your knees pressed back.

3. Straighten your legs part way.

Steps 2 and 3 are 1 set. Do 8 sets.

Keep your pubic bone tucked upward to prevent your back from arching. Abdominals are pulled in, weight is slightly forward, knees are pressed back.

NOTE: Brigitte is a dancer and has a natural turnout. Do not try to turn your toes out this far. Feet slightly turned out or even pointing straight ahead is fine, especially if you have problems with your knees.

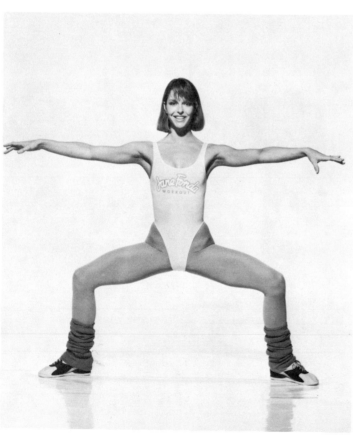

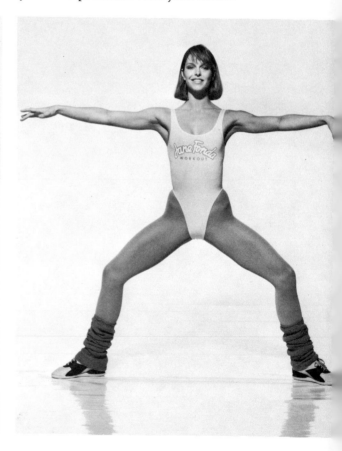

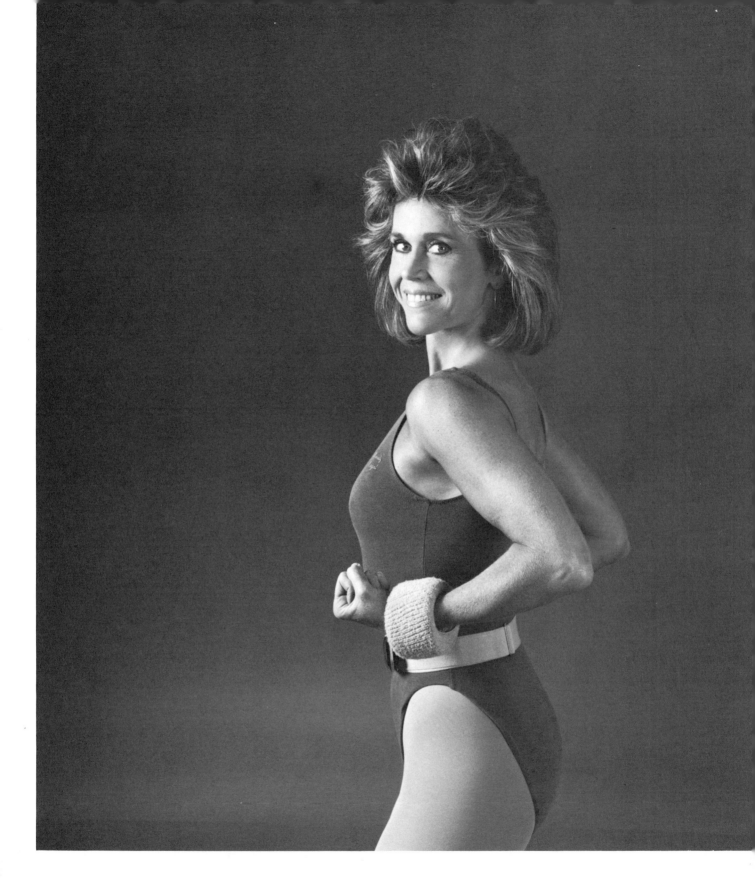

# Upper Body

# 1 · ARM CIRCLES

1. With knees bent and feet parallel (toes pointing forward) bring your arms to the side, shoulder level, and circle your arms *backward* with elbows slightly bent, hands flexed upward. Circle 16 times.

2. Continue circling backward with fists flexed downward, 16 times.

The circling motion is done with the entire arm moving from the shoulder. As the arms move backward, think of pressing your shoulder blades together. Don't let your shoulders hunch up. Knees remain bent.

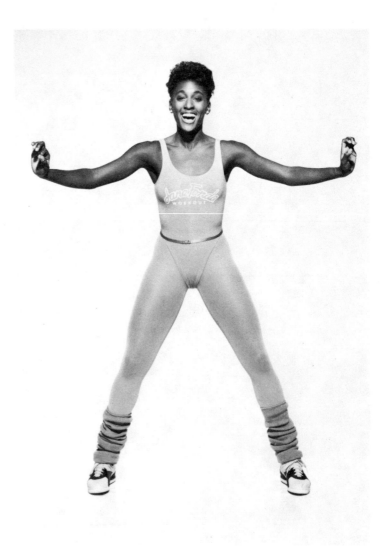

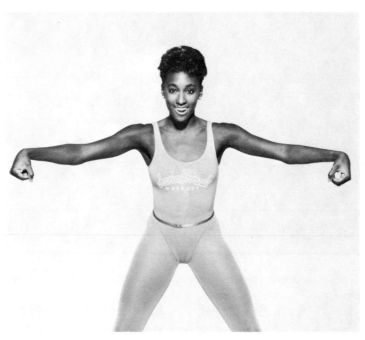

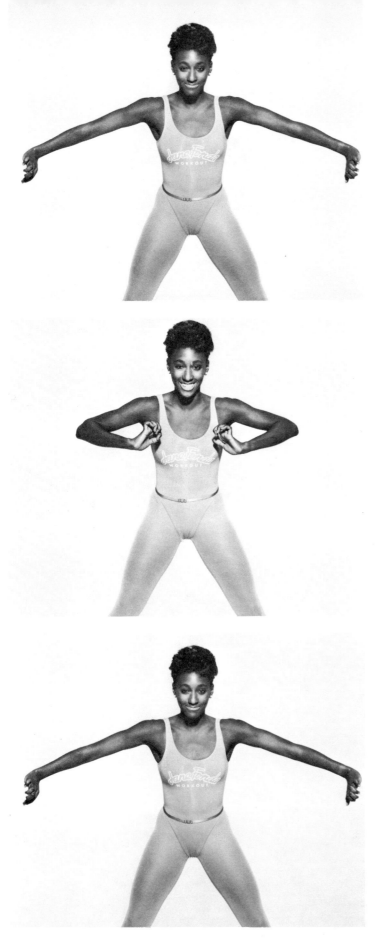

# 2 · ELBOW EXTENSIONS

1. With arms raised to shoulder height, rotate them forward as far as possible in the shoulder socket. The inside of the wrists should be facing upward.

2. Bring your lower arms in toward your body, keeping elbows lifted . . .

3. and extend them out again, resisting the movement as you do.

Steps 2 and 3 are done to 1 count. Repeat for a total of 16 counts.

Keep your elbows at shoulder height. Don't let your shoulders hunch up. Think of making a half circle with your lower arms, always with resistance.

# 3 · SHOULDER TWISTS

1. Extend your arms to the side at shoulder height, palms up.

2. Rotate your arms forward from the shoulders until your palms are facing up again . . .

3. then rotate the arms back again to starting position.

These 2 rotations are 1 set. Do 8 sets.

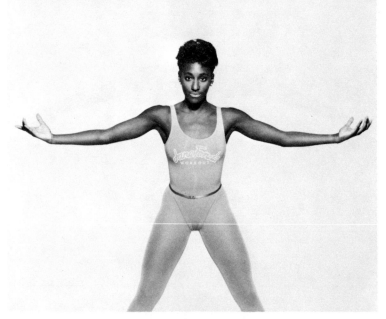

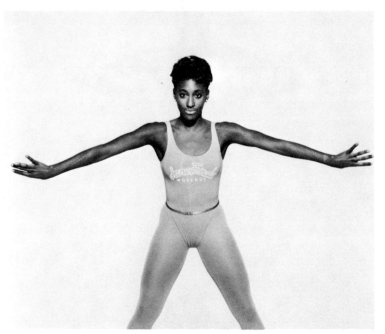

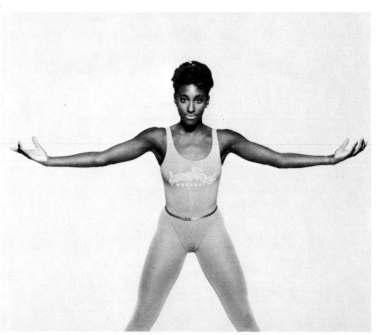

# 4 · BICEPS CURLS

1. Bring your clenched fists in toward your shoulders . . .

2. and extend them out again.

Steps 1 and 2 are done to 1 count. Do 8 counts.

Keep your chest lifted. Resist the inward motion and tighten the biceps muscles.

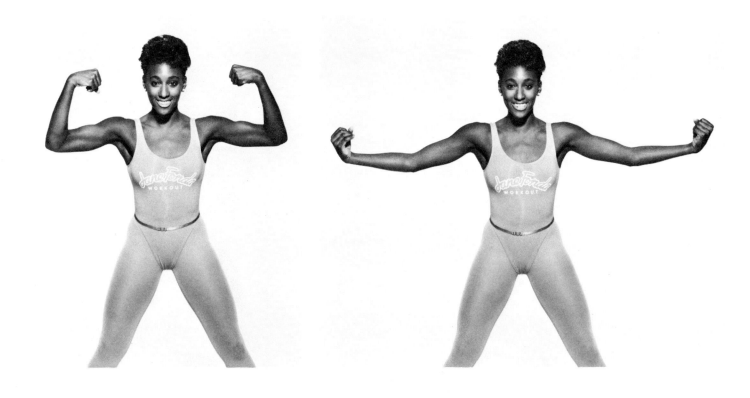

# 5 · PECTORAL PRESSES

1. Keeping both knees slightly bent, bend your elbows at right angles . . .

2. then press your elbows together, resisting the motion.

3. Open them out again.

Press and open to 1 count. Do 8 counts.

As you press inward imagine you are pressing a big beach ball . . . feel the resistance.

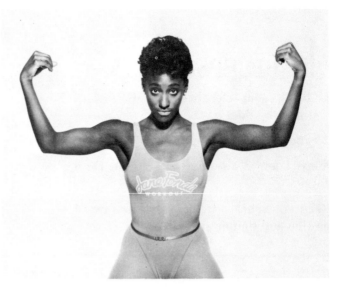

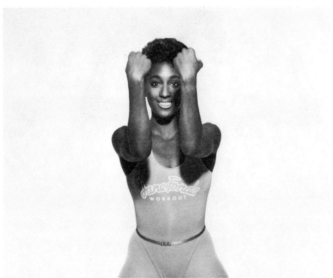

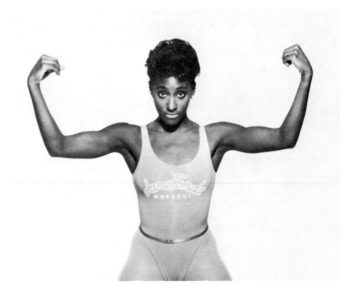

# 6 · TRICEPS EXTENSIONS

1. Keeping your knees bent, bend forward from the hips with your back flat. Elbows are bent up behind you, fists held at the sides of your breasts.

2. Extend your arms backward as high as possible behind your back, with inside of wrists facing downward.

3. Bend arms in again to starting position.

Steps 2 and 3 are done to 1 count. Repeat for 8 counts.

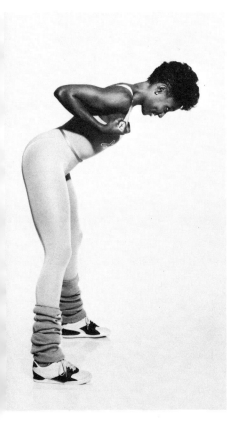
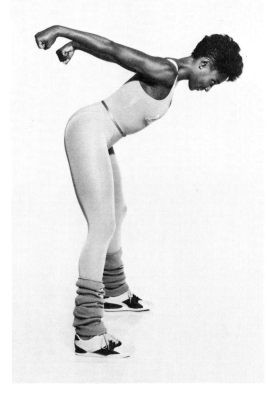
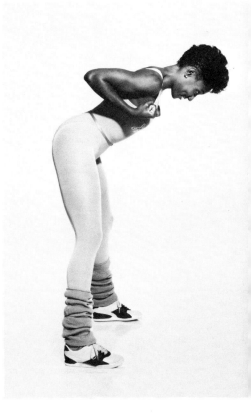

# 7 · DELTOID PRESSES

1. Extend your arms behind your back with hands open, palms facing upward . . .

2. and press them upward 8 times (lowering them a little between each press).

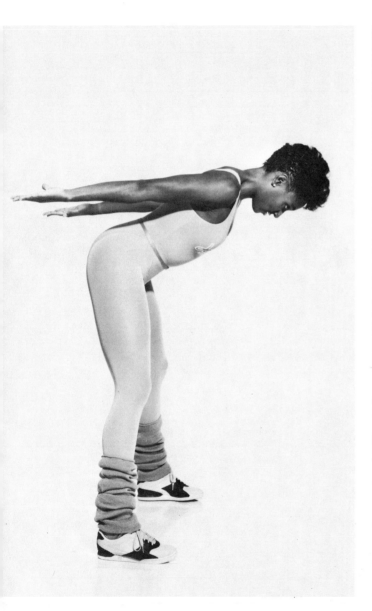
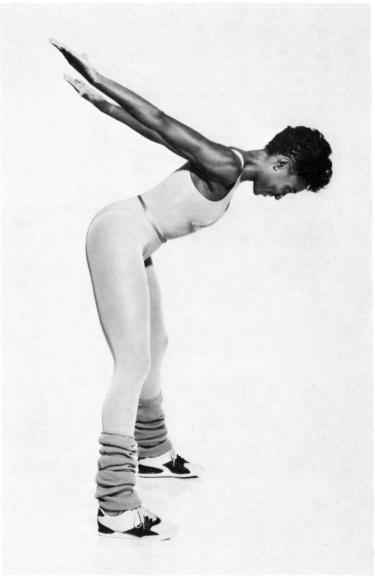

# 8 · SIDE ARM-LIFTS

1. Bring your bent arms down in front of you . . .

2. then lift them out to the side with elbows still slightly bent.

Steps 1 and 2 are done to 1 count. Repeat for a total of 8 counts.

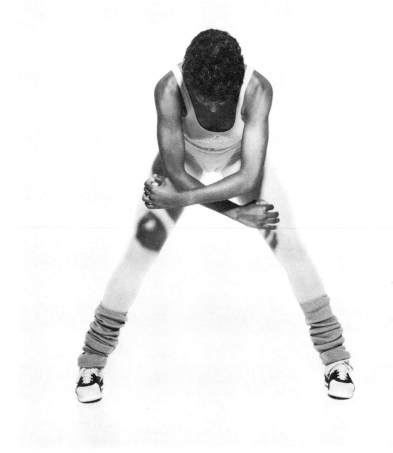

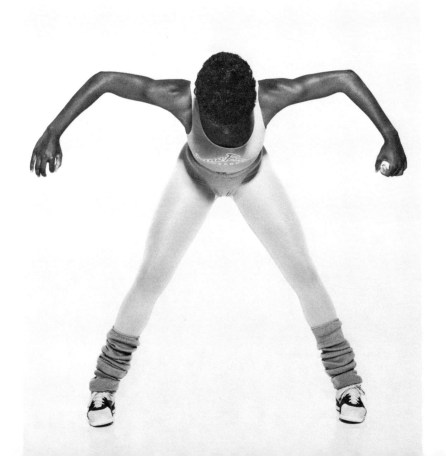

# 9 · SHOULDER STRETCH

1. Standing upright again, bend your right arm behind your head, and press your right elbow downward with your left hand. Hold for 4 long counts.

2. Repeat to the other side. Bend your left arm behind your head and press your left elbow downward with your right hand. Hold for 4 long counts.

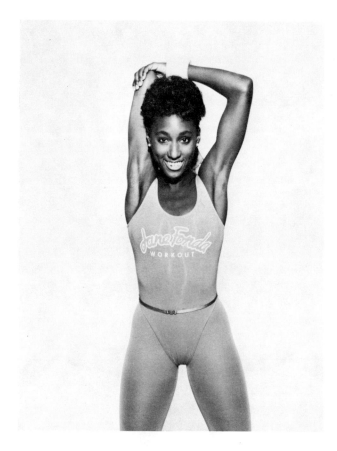 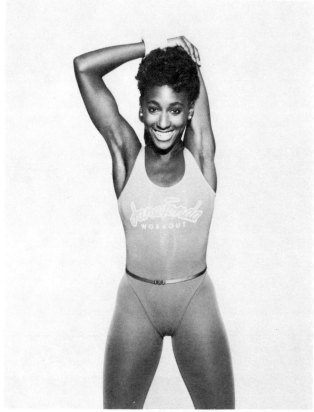

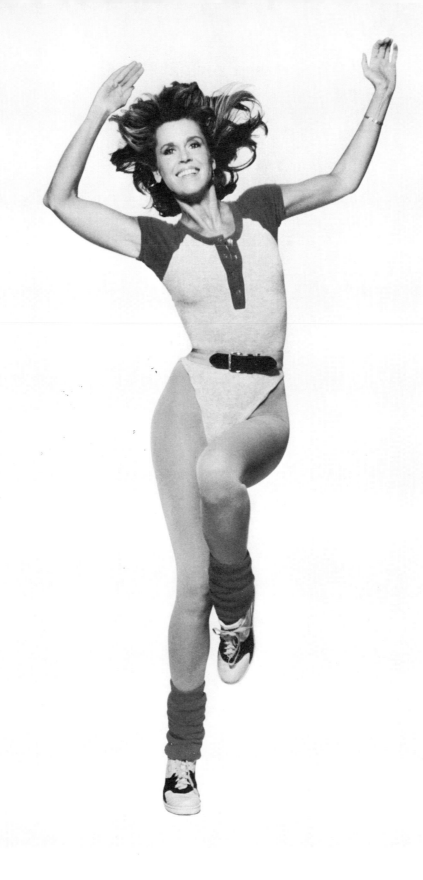

Aerobics

# HOW TO DO IT

Be sure you are wearing good, supportive aerobic shoes.

Put on music that makes you want to move and dance. That's what will motivate you. Your goal is to do 20 to 30 minutes of nonstop aerobic movement.

Start with 5 minutes of small steps in place, lifting your feet only slightly, to gradually raise your pulse rate.

Follow this with 5 minutes of small jogging steps in place. Then begin the more vigorous steps such as skipping, step-kicks, jumping jacks, knee-lifting, can-can kicks, etc. The more you work with your arms overhead, the more you will increase your pulse rate.

To be sure that you are burning stored fat, you should be doing steps that will allow you to carry on a conversation without becoming excessively breathless yet keep your pulse rate within its training zone. At the 15-minute mark, stop and take your pulse. If you are not at your training level push yourself harder by taking larger steps, lifting your knees and legs higher, and doing more of the steps with your arms overhead. (See page 78 for instructions on how to determine your proper training zone.)

The more you vary your steps, the more you will dissipate the stress to your joints and shins. It will also help lessen the impact if you move about over an area at least 3 to 4 feet square as you dance/jog. The more room you have to move about in, the better.

Most important:

---

- Breathe deeply throughout.
- Land on the balls of your feet and allow your heels to touch down.
- Pull up tall. Don't slouch.
- Land with bent knees.
- Don't stop abruptly. Give your heart rate a chance to slow down gradually.

---

Instead of doing 20 to 30 minutes of aerobic dancing to music, you can take a brisk 30- to 40-minute walk, or jog, ride a stationary bike, or do any other aerobic activity. Just be sure to get your cardiovascular work done *at least* 3 to 4 times a week.

# Aerobic Cool-down

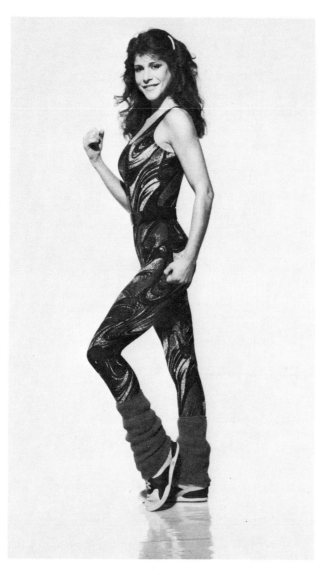

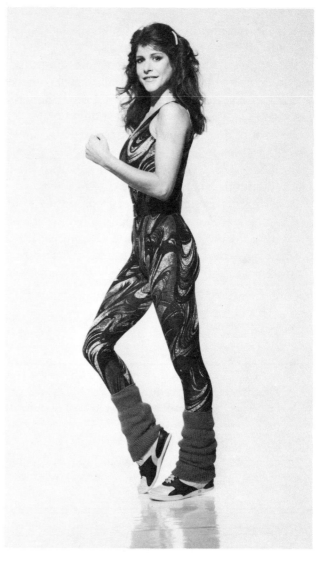

1. For several minutes take prancing steps without jumping . . .

2. . . . while your heart rate begins to slow down and you catch your breath.

3. Then with your legs wide apart, hands on your knees, bend both knees . . .

4. and gently straighten them. Bend and straighten 8 times.

5. Walk your hands on the floor way out in front of you and press your right heel into the floor . . .

6. then press the left heel into the floor. Pressing right and left is 1 set. Do 8 sets.

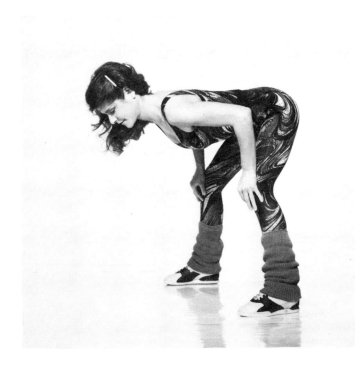 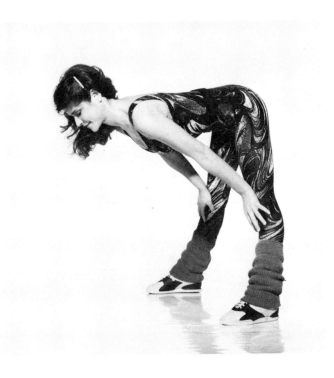

Abdominals are pulled in, hips are stretching toward the ceiling, pubic bone is curling toward your navel.

*(continued)*

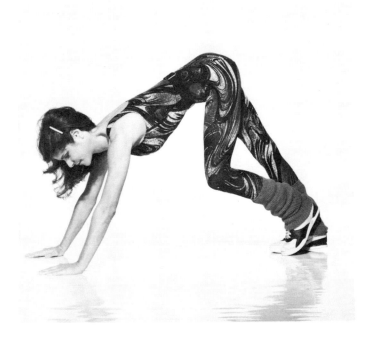 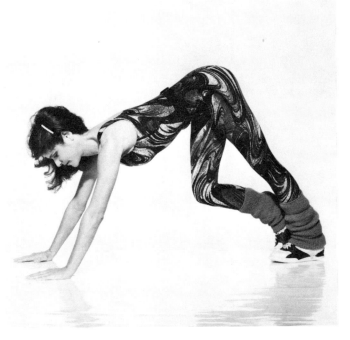

7. Walk your feet toward your hands, bend your knees, round your back . . .

8. and slowly roll up, one vertebra at a time . . .

9. to a standing position.

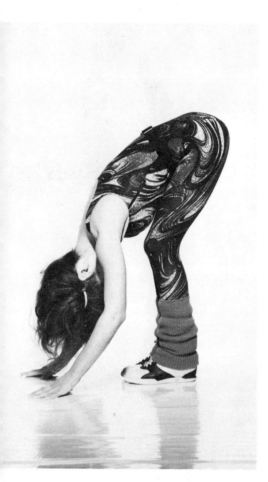 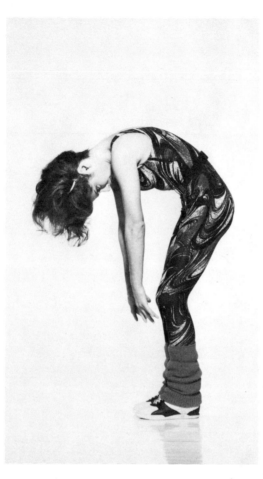 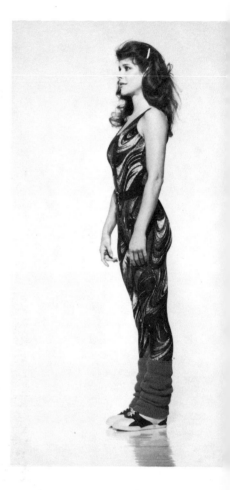

*Get yourself a towel, folded blanket, or mat and we'll go on to floor work.*

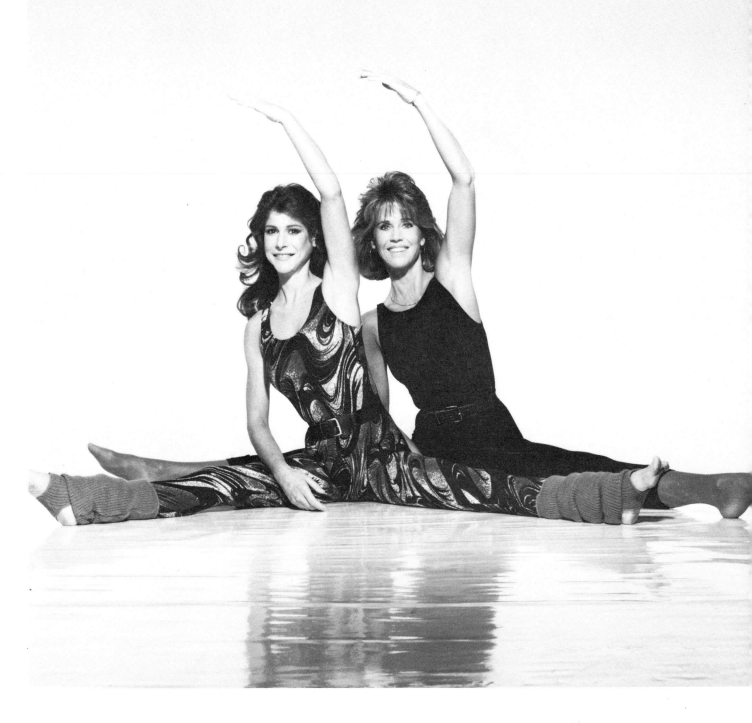

# Floor Stretch

*You should remove your shoes now. These stretches should be done on a mat or blanket to cushion your hips and back and keep dust out of your nose and hair.*

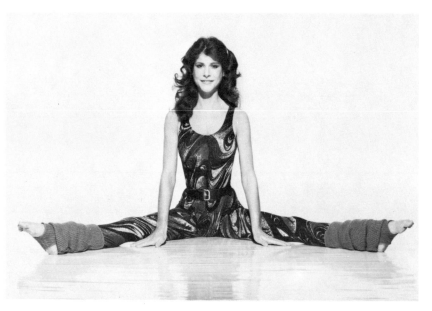

# 1 · FLOOR STRETCH

1. Sitting on the floor, open your legs as wide as you can without straining. Point your toes.

2. Pull over to the right side. Your left arm is reaching directly over your head to the right. Press your left shoulder back. Hold for 16 counts, continuing to stretch and lengthen the left side. Don't bounce.

3. Turn and face your right leg, hands on either side of it. Reach out over that leg with your torso for 8 counts. Press your left hip into the floor.

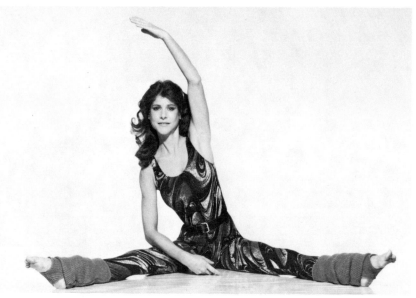

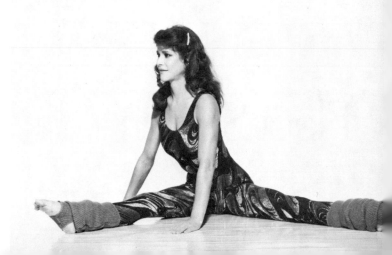

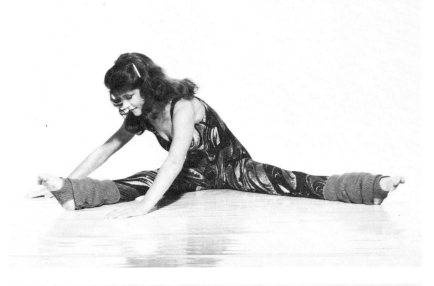

4. Round your back and pull down over your right leg. Stretch and breathe for 8 counts.

5. Roll torso back up to center position, then . . .

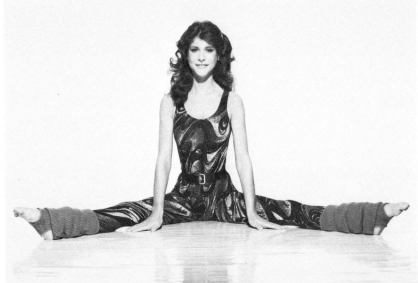

6. repeat to the left, pulling over to the side with your right arm reaching directly overhead. Press your right shoulder back. Hold for 16 counts, stretching and lengthening the right side. Don't bounce.

*(continued)*

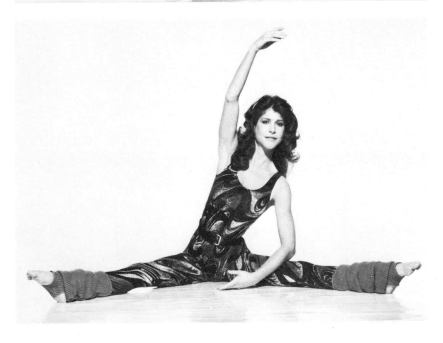

7. Turn and face your left leg. Reach out over that leg with your torso for 8 counts. Press your right hip into the floor.

8. Round your back and pull down over your left leg. Stretch and breathe for 8 counts.

9. With your hands on the floor in front of you, "walk" yourself to the center, flex your feet, and stretch out over the floor, lengthening your spine for 16 counts.

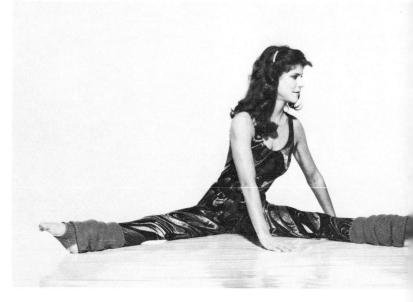

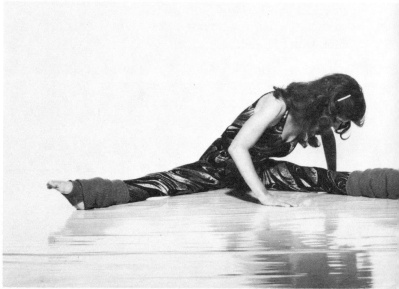

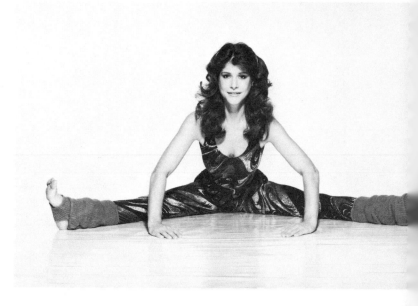

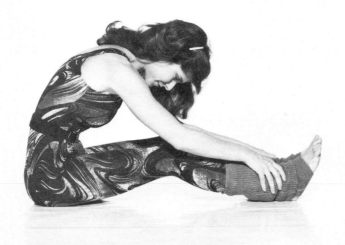

# 2 · HAMSTRING STRETCH

1. Bring your legs together in front of you with feet flexed and knees slightly bent. Round your head and torso down over your legs and hold for 12 counts. Don't hold your breath.

2. Bend your knees more, pull in your abdominals, and roll up to a sitting position.

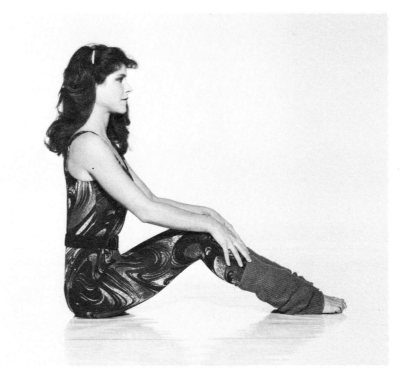

*Now roll onto your back and go right into the abdominal work.*

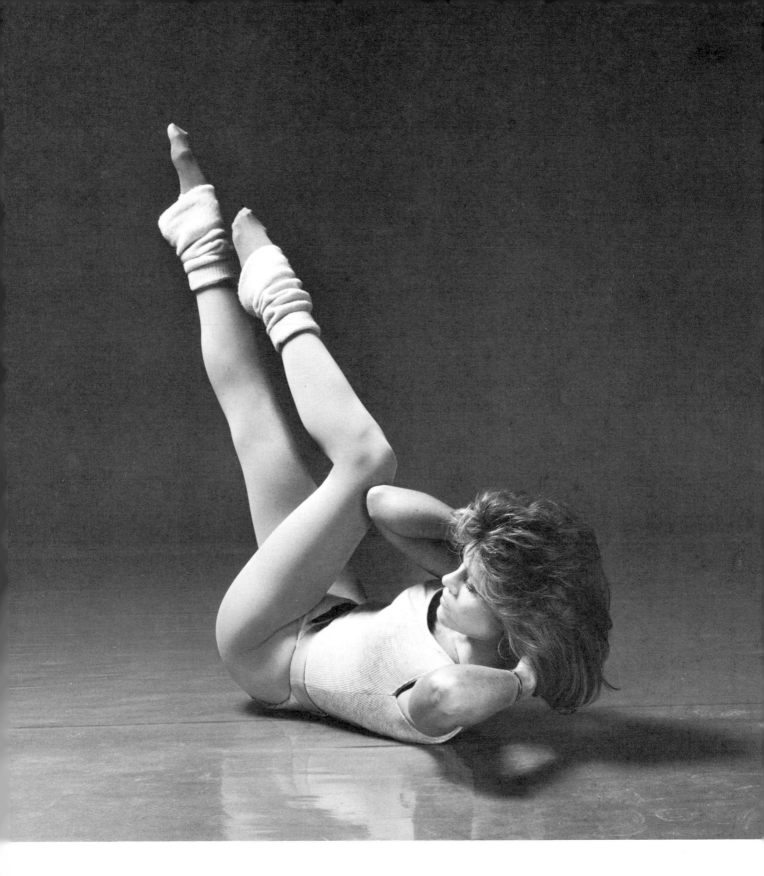

# Abdominals

*We've pretty much finished the fat-burning portion of the Workout. Now we'll begin the muscle-building that will raise our basal metabolism.*

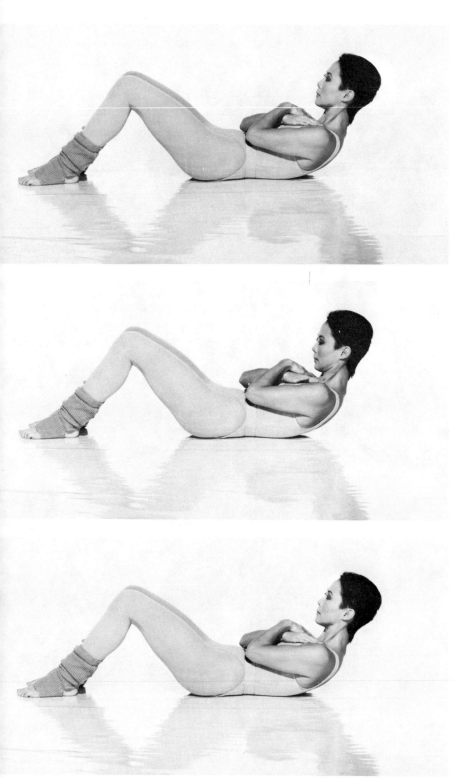

# 1 · SLOW CURLS

1. Lie on your back, knees bent, feet about hip-distance apart. Arms are crossed on your chest. Tuck your chin in, inhale, and . . .

2. slowly curl up, raising shoulders off the floor, for 3 counts. Exhale as you curl up.

3. Inhale as you release back several inches.

The curl-up and release are 1 set. Do 4 sets.

EXHALE AS YOU CURL UP. INHALE AS YOU RELEASE.

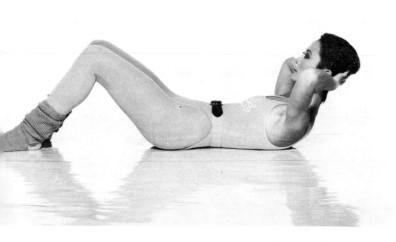

# $2 \cdot$ SIT-UPS

1. Lie flat on the floor, hands behind your head, elbows out to the side. Lift your head and shoulders off the floor as high as you can . . .

2. then lower a little but do not touch the floor.

Lift and lower 20 times without letting shoulders touch the floor.

EXHALE AS YOU LIFT. INHALE AS YOU LOWER.

All the lifting is done with the abdominals, not the arms. Don't put pressure on your neck with your hands.

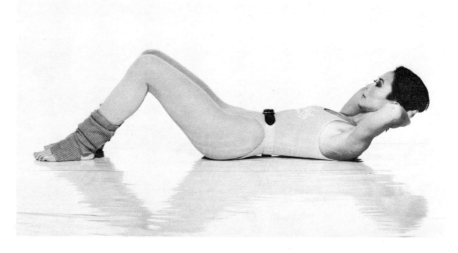

# 3 · CRUNCHES

1. Lift your legs, cross your ankles and bend your knees slightly. Hands behind your head with elbows pointing forward.

2. Reach up toward your knees with your upper body, then release back slightly.

Reach and release 24 times.

EXHALE AS YOU REACH; INHALE AS YOU RELEASE.

The movement is very small. Try to keep your shoulder blades off the floor, even when you release. Use your abdominals to raise your upper body, not your arms.

Without breaking rhythm go right on to . . .

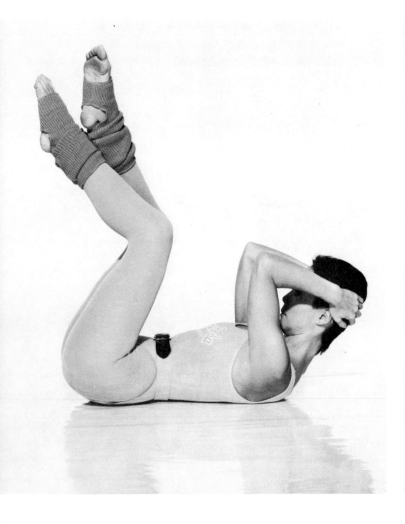 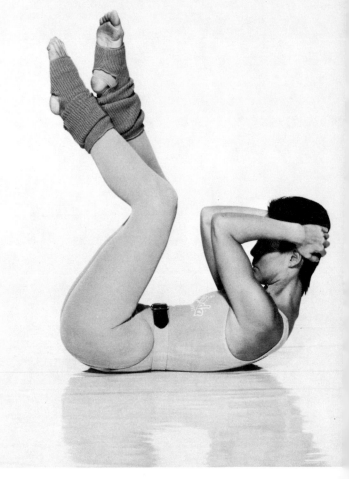

# 4 · CROSSOVERS

1. Reach your right elbow across to the outside of your left knee . . .

2. . . . then, trying not to let the shoulders release back very much, reach your left elbow to the outside of your right knee.

Reaching right and left is 1 set. Do 16 sets.

These movements work the oblique muscles along the side of the waist.

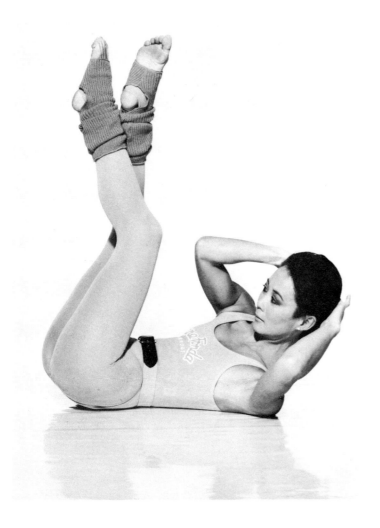
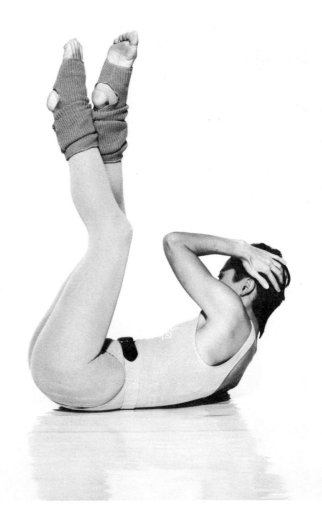

# 5 · HIP STRETCH

1. Relax your head and neck. Clasp your
   hands behind your knees and hug your
   knees to your chest.

TAKE A DEEP BREATH, THEN EXHALE.

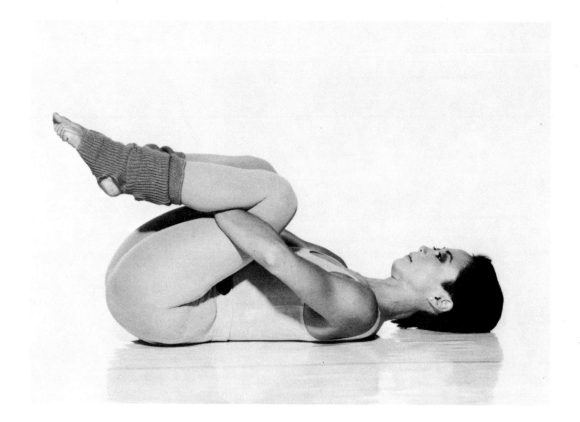

# 6 · MORNING STAR

Extend your left leg straight out on the floor. Bend your right knee, cross it over the left, and press it down toward the floor on the left side with your left hand. Be sure to curl your pubic bone up toward your navel. Your right arm is extended straight out to the side from the shoulder. Try to press your right shoulder to the floor. Hold for 8 counts.

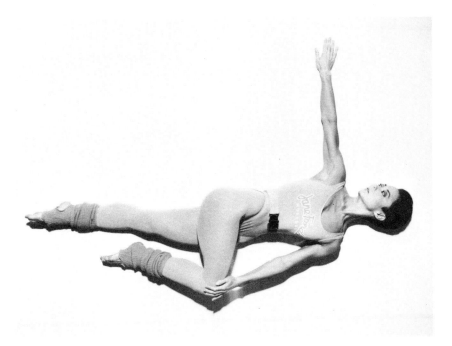

Repeat to the left: your right leg is extended straight out on the floor. Bend your left knee, cross it over the right, and press it down toward the floor on the right side with your right hand. Again, the pubic bone is curled up toward your navel. Your left arm is extended straight out to the side from the shoulder. Press your left shoulder to the floor. Hold for 8 counts.

This exercise stretches the abdominals, the hips, and the shoulder, and it decompresses the spine.

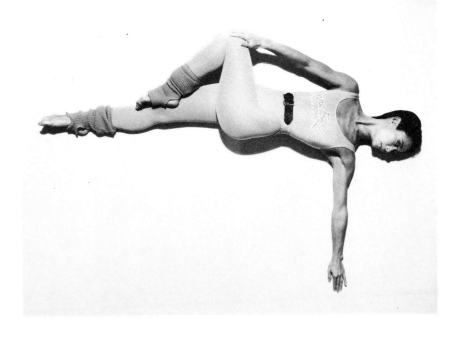

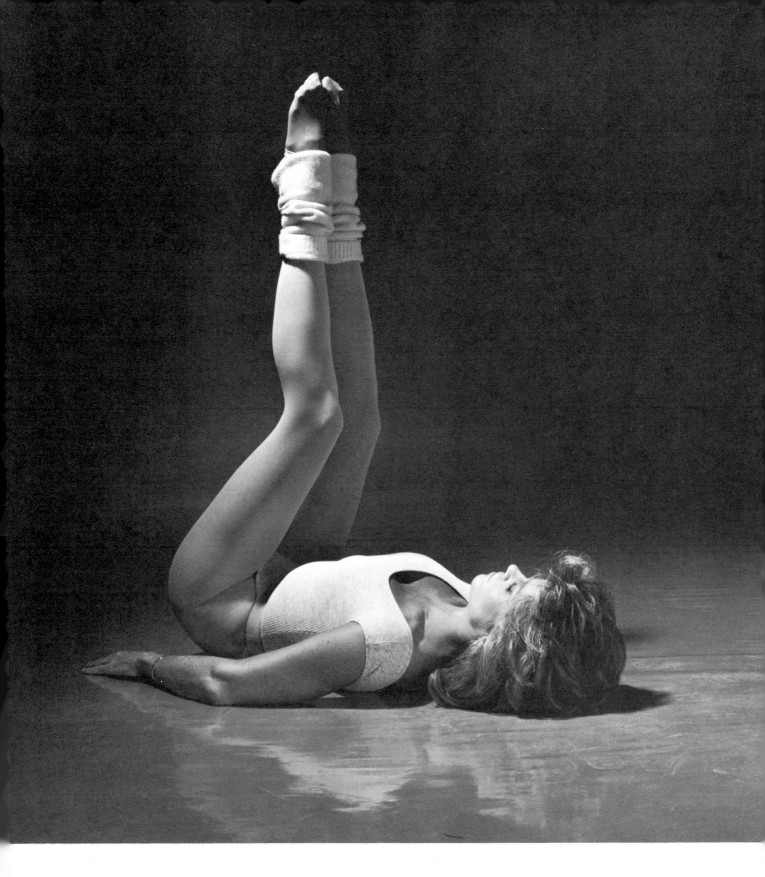

# Legs and Hips

*Go through all the leg and hip exercises using your right leg, as illustrated. When you finish the series repeat each exercise using the left leg.*

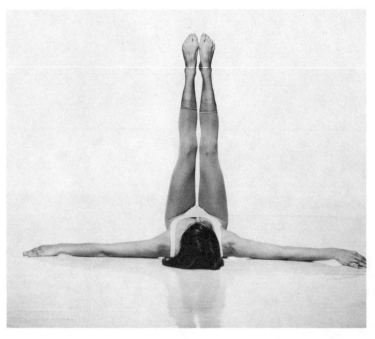

# 1 · INNER THIGHS

1. Lie on your back, arms out to the side, legs straight up in the air, toes pointed.

2. Open your legs wide . . .

3. and flex your feet as you bring your legs together and cross one over the other.

Steps 2 and 3 are 1 set. Do 12 sets, alternating the leg that closes in front.

Resist the closing of the legs so that you really work that inner thigh muscle.

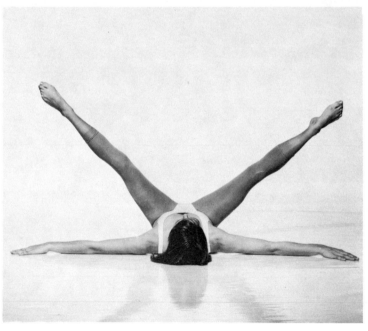

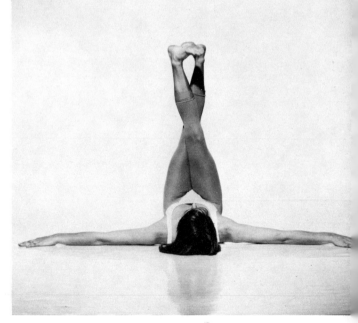

# $2 \cdot$ PARALLEL LEG LIFTS

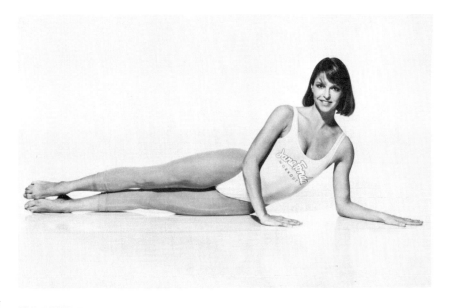

1. Lie on your left side, up on your elbow with palms flat on the floor. Extend both legs straight out on a line with your torso.

2. Point your toes and slowly lift your right leg as high as you can with your right hip pressing forward.

3. Slowly lower your leg part way. Don't let it touch your bottom leg.

Lift and lower 12 times.

*Be sure your top hip is pressing forward;* don't rock back. Keep leg stretched out long as you lift it. Don't sink into your shoulder; lengthen the torso.

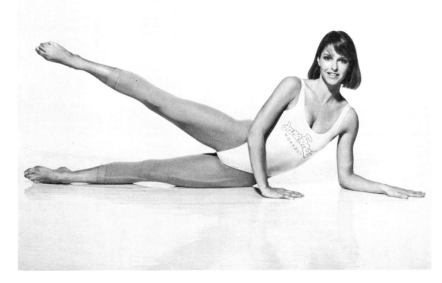

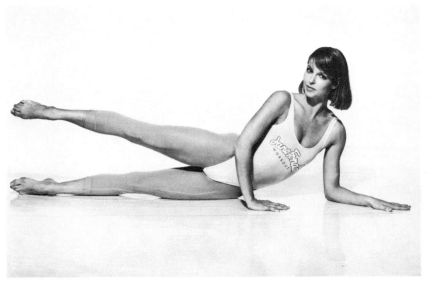

# $3 \cdot$ LEG LIFTS

1. Bend your bottom knee and bring it out in front of you. Flex your right foot.

2. In a faster tempo lift your right leg . . .

3. and lower it part way.

Lift and lower 12 times.

Keep your weight forward on the hand in front of you.

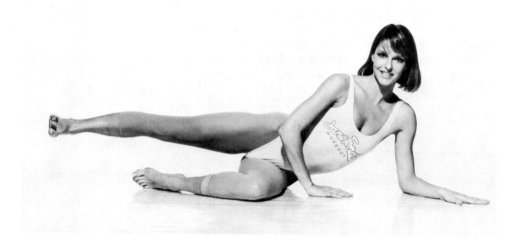

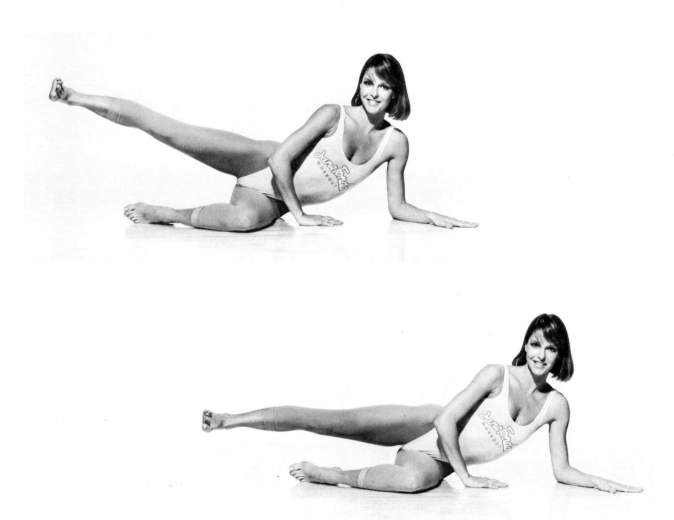

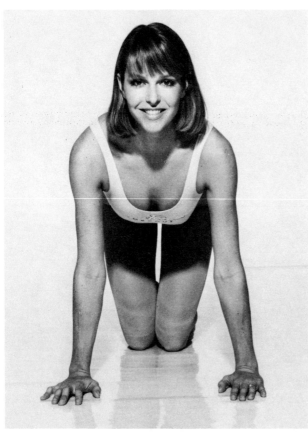

# 4 · ROVER'S REVENGE

1. On your hands and knees with weight evenly distributed, your stomach pulled in, pubic bone curled toward your navel . . .

2. lift your bent right knee out to the side to hip height . . .

3. then lower your knee almost to the floor.

Lift and lower 16 times.

4. Then do 8 small lifts from a raised position . . .

5. lowering the knee just a few inches between lifts.

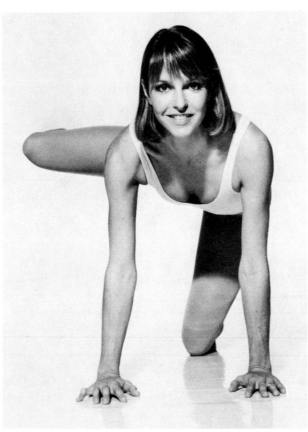

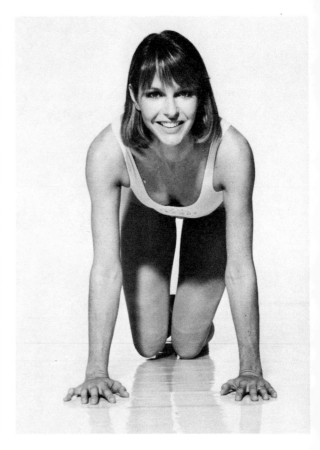

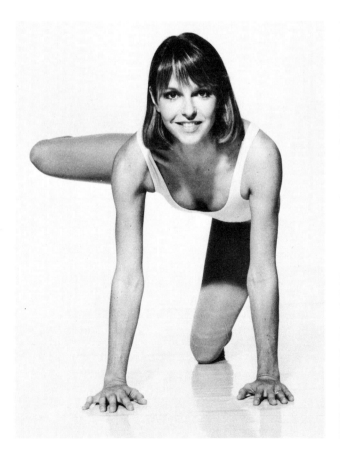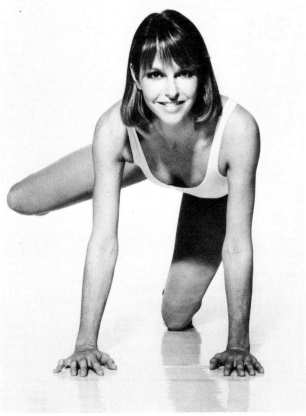

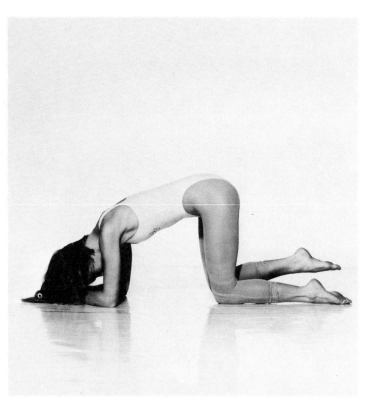

# 5 · BENT LEG LIFTS

1. Come down onto your elbows, head down, and with pointed toes and buttocks squeezed tight . . .

2. lift your bent right leg behind you as high as you can without straightening it . . .

3. and lower your leg again, knee almost to the floor.

Lift and lower 16 times.

EXHALE AS YOU LIFT. INHALE AS YOU LOWER.

Don't let your back arch as you lift your leg. Keep your buttocks squeezed tight and your pubic bone tucked toward your navel. Your leg should lift against the resistance of your contracted buttock muscles.

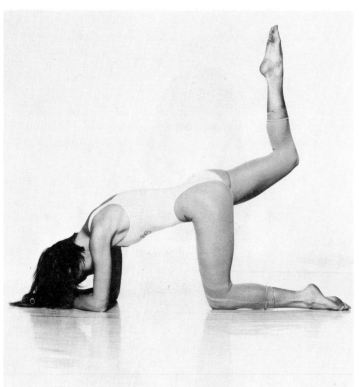

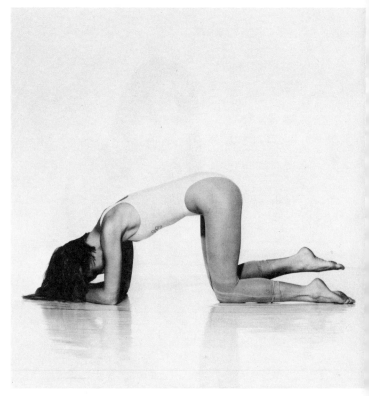

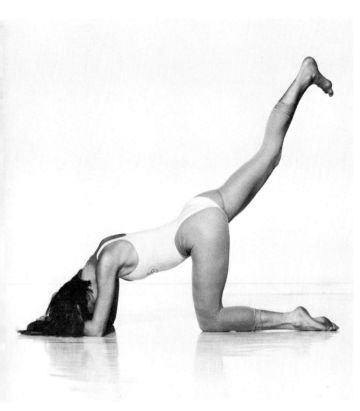

# 6 · DONKEY KICKS

1. Extend your right leg high up behind you. Flex your foot, squeeze your buttocks tight, and curl your pubic bone toward your navel to keep your back from arching.

2. Bend your flexed foot in toward your buttocks, keeping your knee lifted as high as possible.

3. Extend your leg again, lifting it higher.

Bend in and extend 8 times.

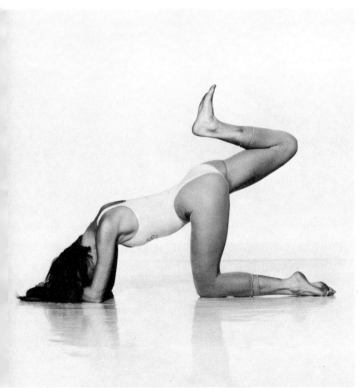

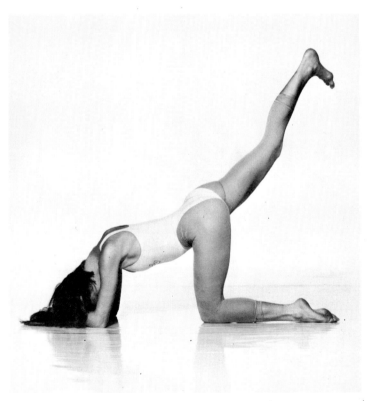

# 7 · LEG EXTENSIONS

1. Point your toes and extend your right leg as high as possible. Squeeze the buttocks and hold 8 counts, extending and lifting the leg as you do.

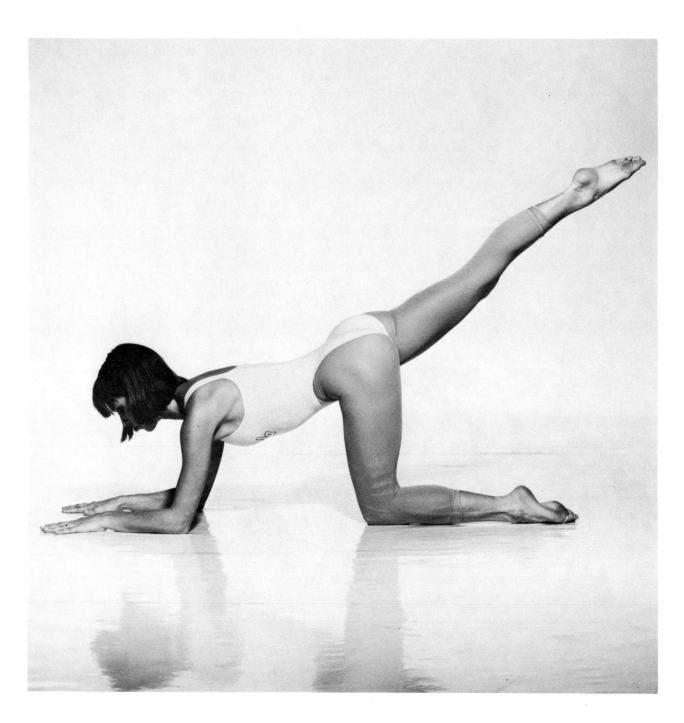

# 8 · TAILOR POSITION

1. Cross your right leg (the one you've been working) in front of your left leg.

2. Round down over your *left* knee. Relax and breathe. Feel the stretch in the right hip.

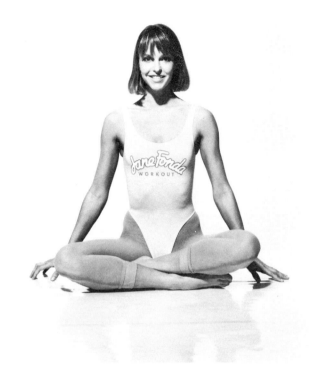

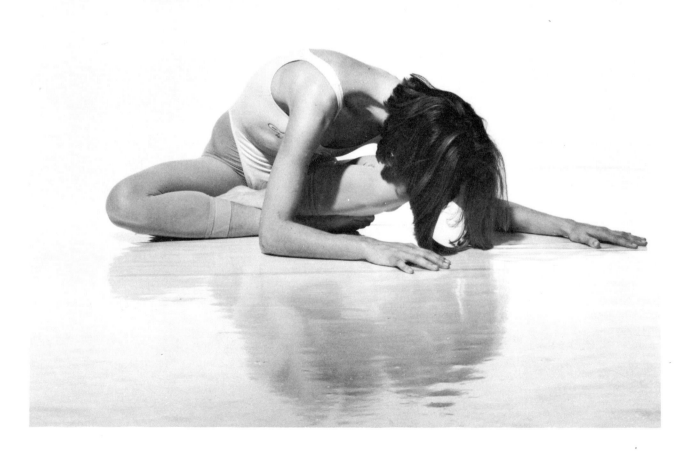

# 9 · TORSO STRETCH

1. Sit up and straighten your left leg. Wrap your left arm around your bent right knee and gently press the knee to your chest. Your back is straight, your right palm is flat on the floor behind your back. Look over your right shoulder and breathe deeply.

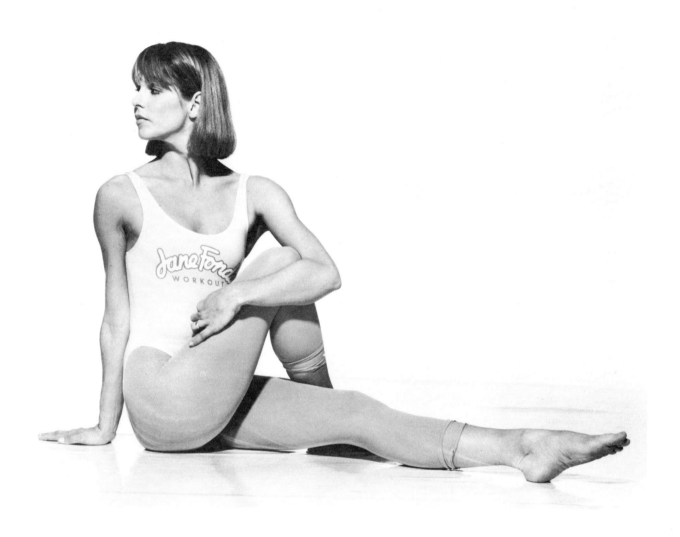

*Now we'll repeat all the leg and hip exercises, starting with the Parallel Leg Lifts, working the left leg.*

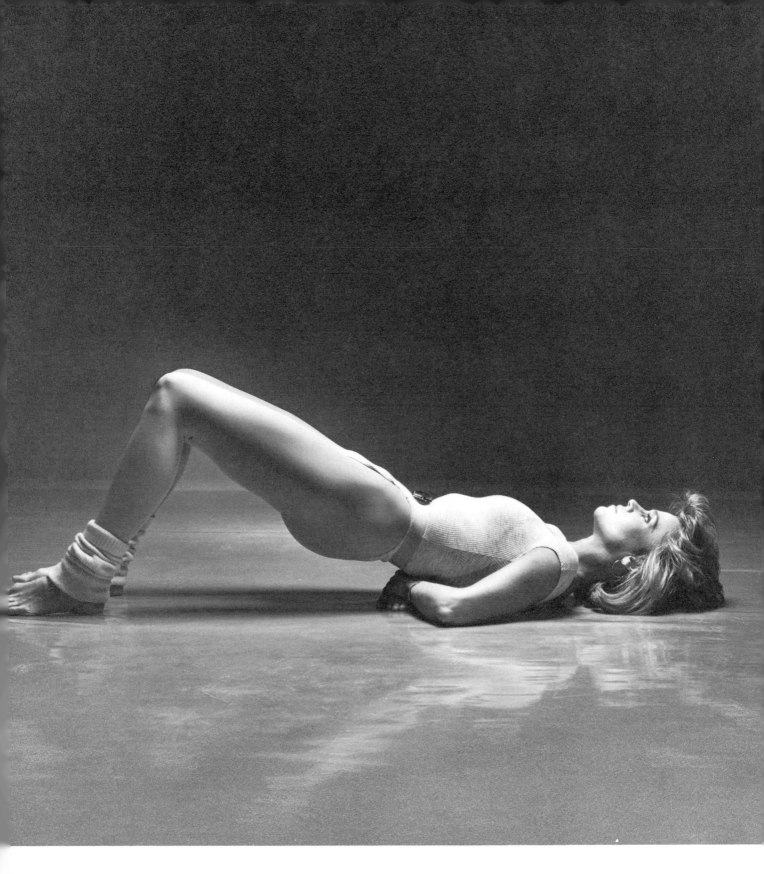

# Buttocks

# 1 · PELVIC CURLS

These movements are very small but intense. Your hips may move only a few inches.

1. Lie on your back, feet and knees parallel, a little more than hip-distance apart. Place one hand on top of the other, palms down, directly beneath your lower back, which should touch your hands at all times.

2. Curl your pubic bone upward toward your navel, squeezing your buttock muscles as you do . . .

3. then relax these muscles a little.

Do steps 2 and 3 slowly 16 times and faster 16 times.

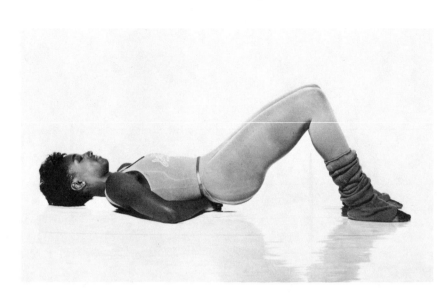

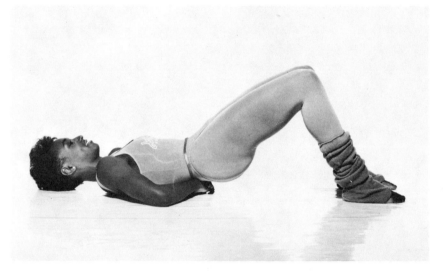

# 2 · KNEE PRESSES

1. Move your feet a little farther apart. With pubic bone curled upward, bring your knees apart . . .

2. and together, squeezing your buttock muscles even tighter as you bring knees together.

Steps 1 and 2 are done to 1 count. Do 16 counts slowly, then 16 counts faster, while keeping your buttocks tightly squeezed.

Resist the movement of your knees coming together. This should work your inner thigh muscles as well as your buttocks. Think of bringing the upper part of the inner thighs, the part closest to the buttocks, together first.

*Do not let your back arch.*

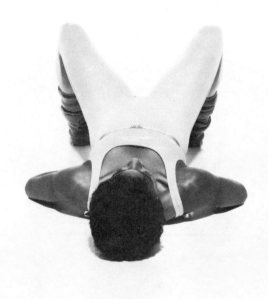 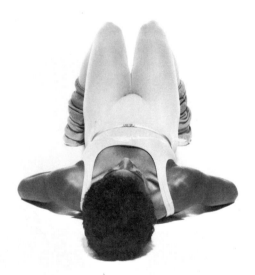

# 3 · BURN-OUT

1. Press your knees toward each other (they don't have to touch), then curl your buttocks upward and release them slightly for 16 times.

Keep your lower back touching your hands. You should feel it deep inside the buttock muscles.

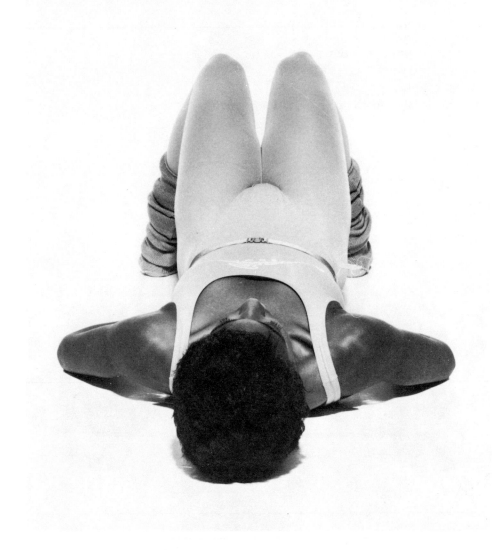

*Go right into the Cool-down without stopping.*

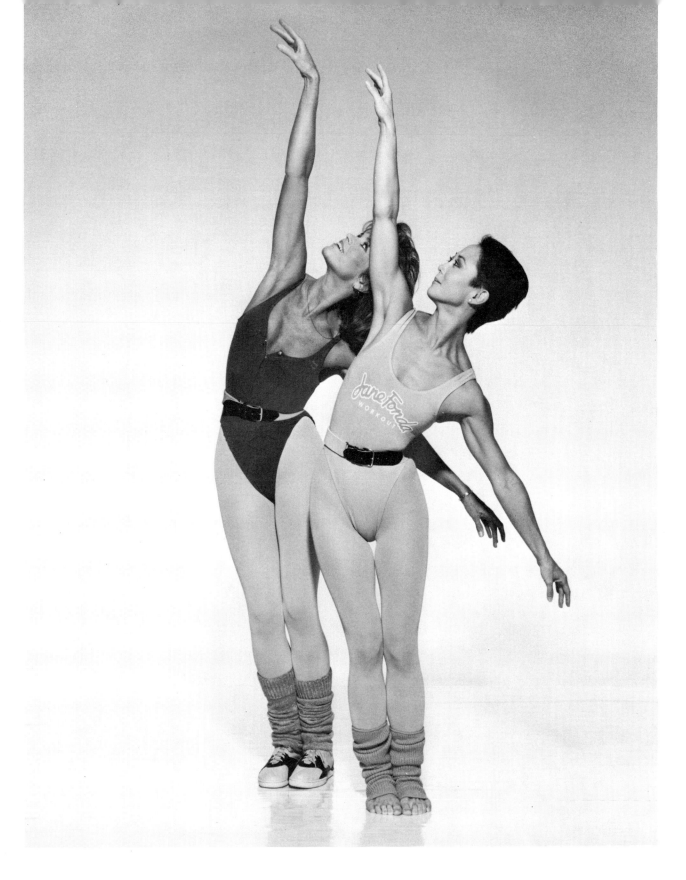

# Cool-down

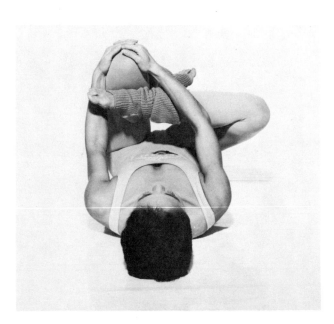

# 1 · HIP AND HAMSTRING STRETCH

1. Place your right ankle against your left knee and with your hands pull your left knee to your chest, stretching the right hip. Hold for 8 counts.

2. Place your left foot on the floor and stretch that right leg straight up, pressing it gently toward your chest with toes pointed . . .

3. then flexed.

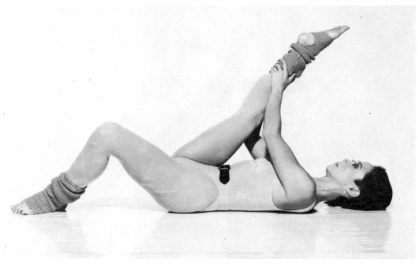

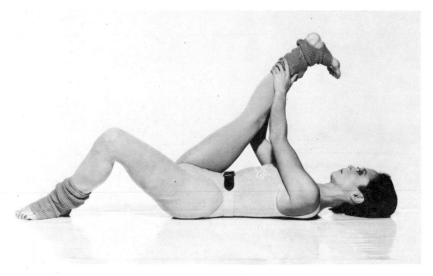

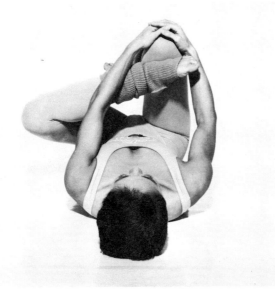

4. Place your left ankle against your right knee and with your hands pull your right knee to your chest, stretching the left hip. Hold for 8 counts.

5. Place your right foot on the floor and stretch that left leg straight up, pressing it gently toward your chest with toes pointed . . .

6. then flexed.

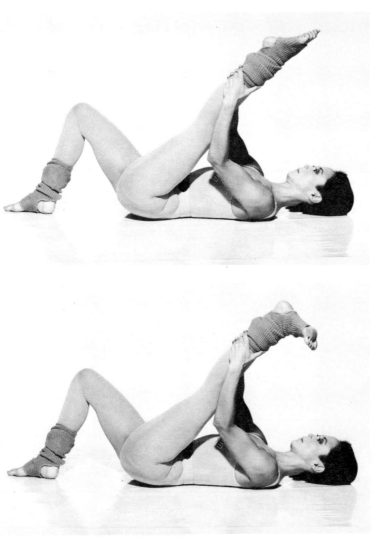

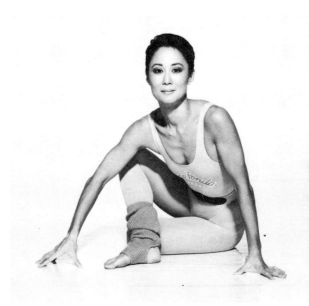

Roll up to a sitting position and bring one leg across the other. With foot flat on floor push off and come to a standing position with feet apart.

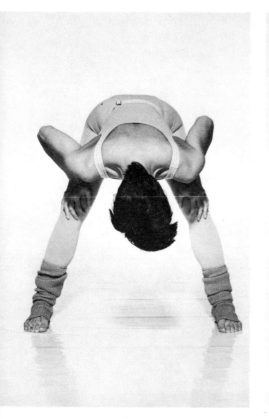
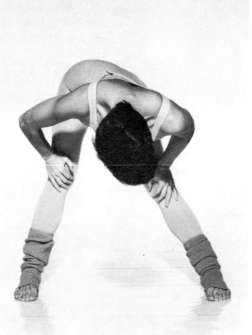
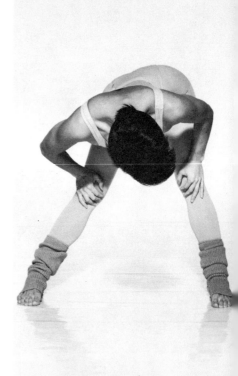

# 2 · GROIN STRETCH

1. Let your upper body drop down over your straight legs with hands on your thighs or knees.

2. Press your hips to the right . . .

3. and to the left.

Feel a stretch in the groin. Repeat once on each side, then bend your knees and roll up.

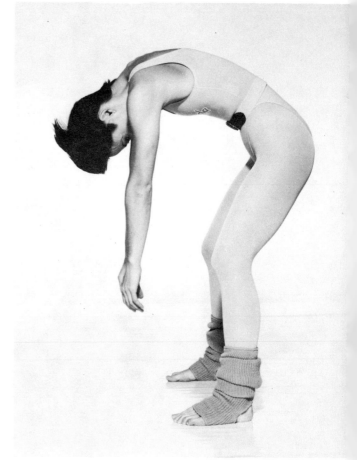

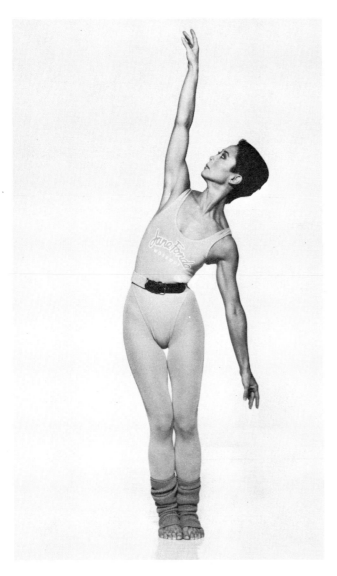 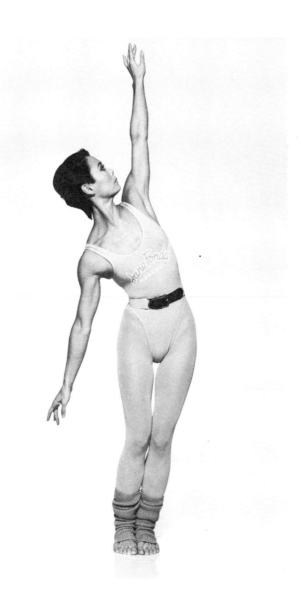

# 3 · SIDE STRETCH

1. Bring your feet together, knees bent. Reach up with your right arm and down with your left arm. Twist your torso slightly toward the raised arm. Look up toward the raised arm and feel a stretch up that side. Knees stay bent.

2. Repeat to the other side, reaching up with your left arm and down with your right arm. Look up toward your raised left arm and feel a stretch up that side. Knees stay bent.

**GOOD GOING! KEEP IT UP!**

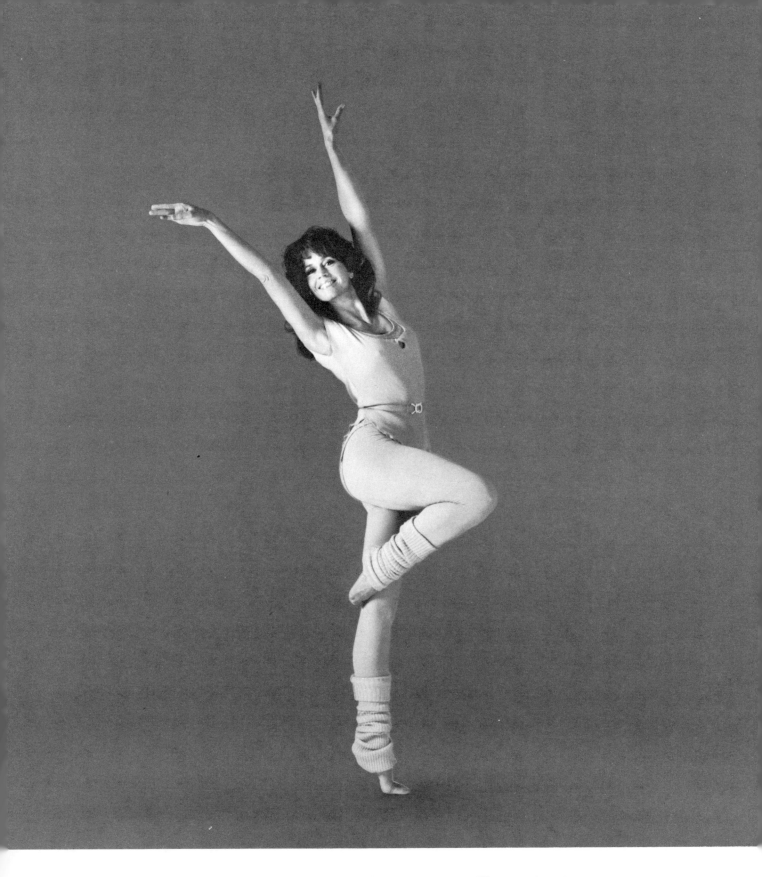

# ADVANCED WORKOUT

*Move smoothly in time to the music from one exercise to the next. Concentrate on doing the movements correctly and making the muscles work deeply. Don't just go through the motions.*

**Correct Standing Posture:**

*Curl your pubic bone up toward your navel. Stomach should be pulled in, chest is lifted, shoulders are pressed back and down. Weight is slightly forward.*

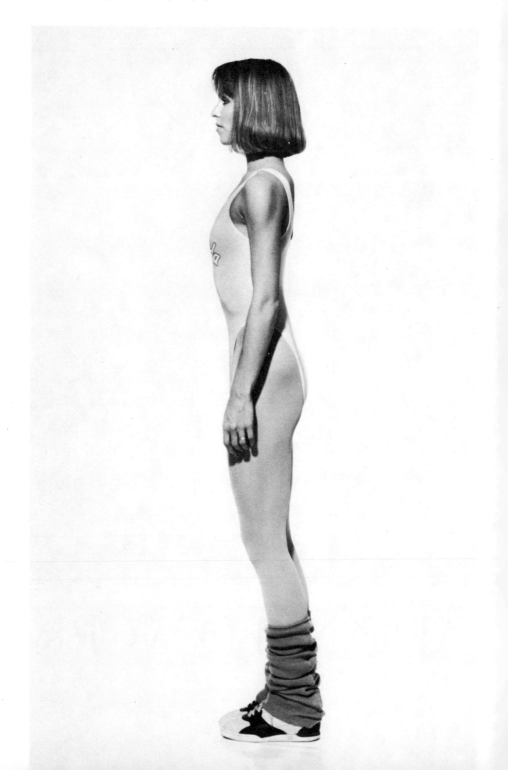

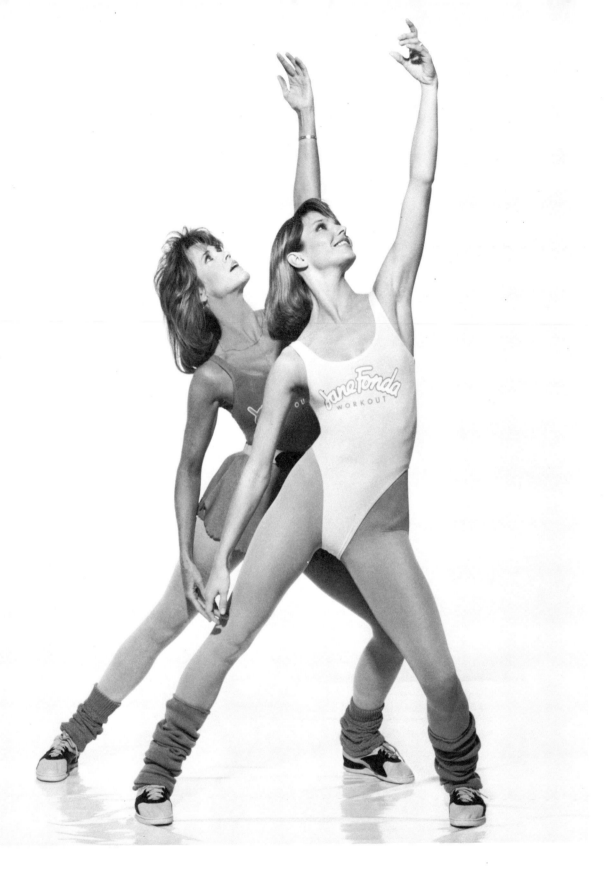

# Warm-up

*Starting Position: Pull up tall from the waist, buttocks squeezed tight, stomach in, knees slightly bent, feet parallel a little more than hip-distance apart. Shoulders are pressed back and down.*

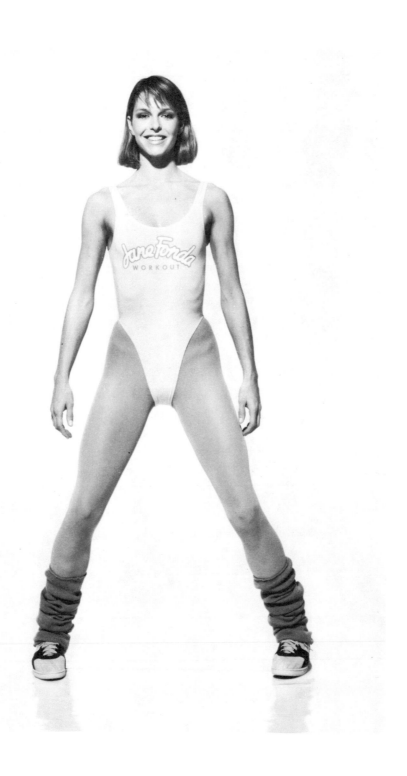

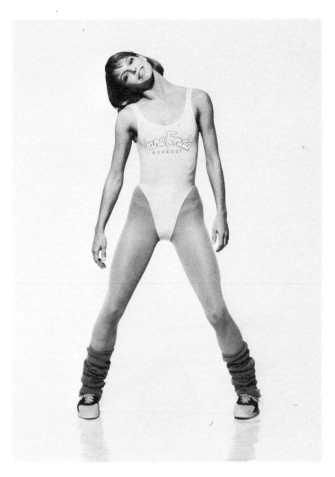

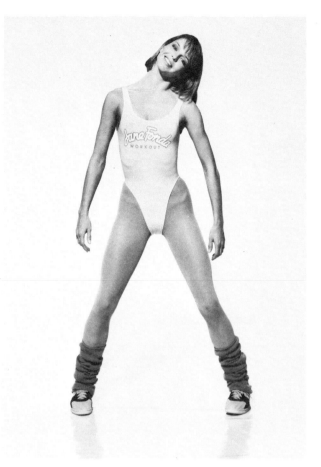

# 1 · HEAD PRESSES

1. Press your right ear toward your right shoulder and stretch for 4 counts. Feel the stretch in the left side of your neck. Be sure your shoulders are pressed back and down.

2. Press your left ear toward your left shoulder and stretch for 4 counts.

Repeat 4 counts to the right, 4 counts to the left.

3. Bring your head back to center.

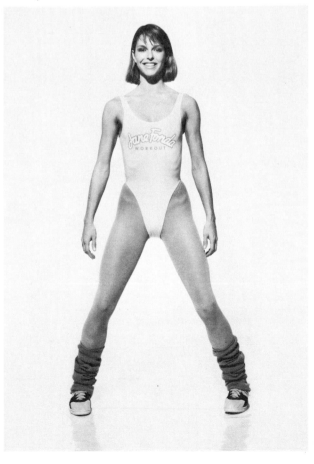

# 2 · SHOULDER ROLLS

1. Lift your shoulders up toward your ears and circle them backward . . .

2. and down again in a big circle. Do 8 slow circles.

Be sure to get full motion in your shoulders and to keep your stomach pulled in, pubic bone tucked up, and weight slightly forward. Knees are still bent.

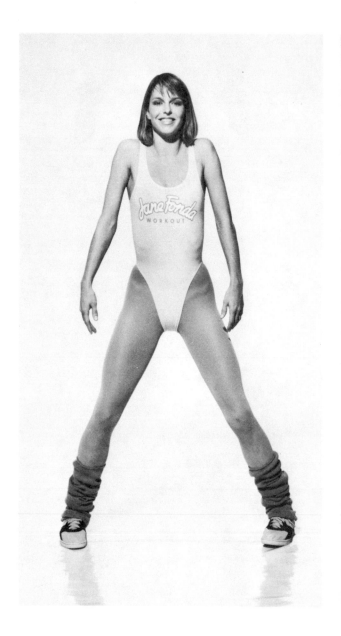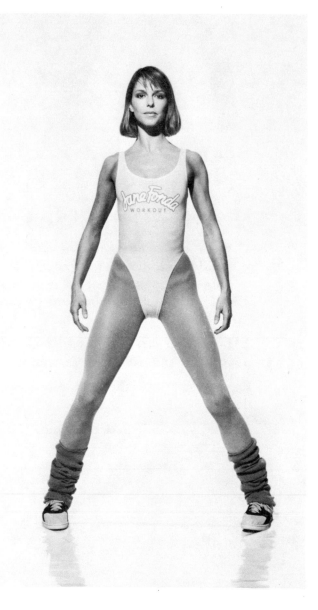

# 3 · ELBOW CIRCLES

1. Keep your knees slightly bent. Place your hands on your shoulders, lift your elbows to the sides at shoulder height, and circle your elbows forward and up . . .

2. then down and back 16 times.

Think of pressing your shoulder blades together as your elbows circle backward.

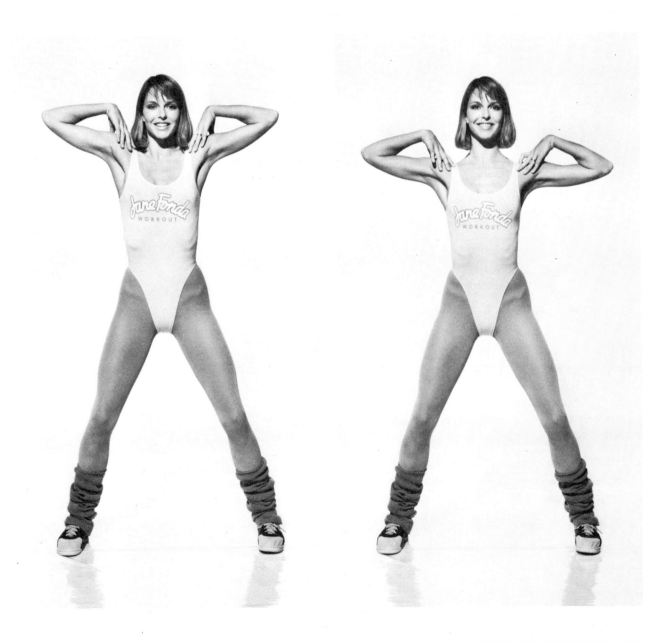

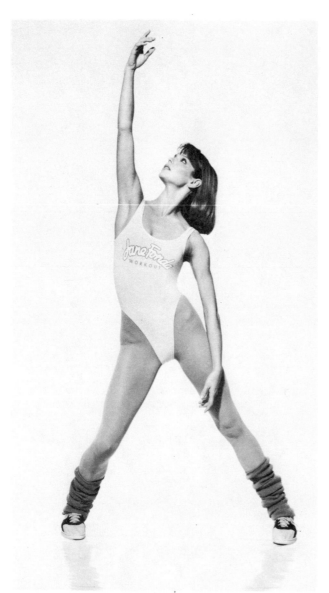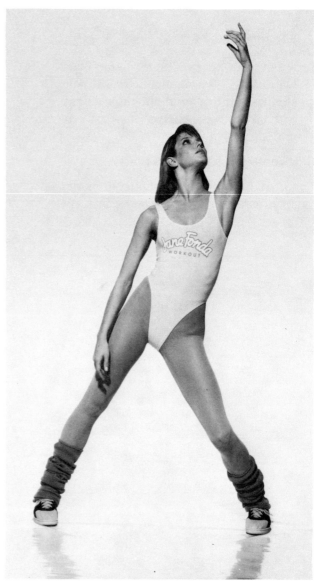

# 4 · WAIST LIFTS

1. With feet parallel, stretch your right arm upward as you bend your right knee. Feel a stretch up your right side.

2. Stretch your left arm upward as you bend your left knee. Feel a stretch up your left side.

Stretching right and left is 1 set. Do 8 sets.

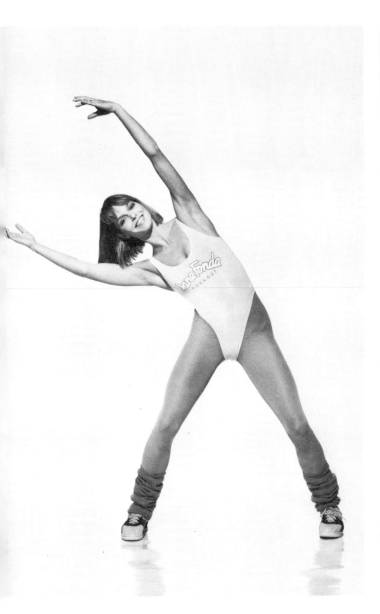
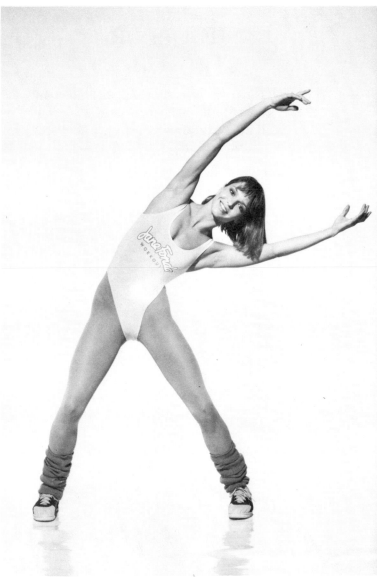

# 5 · WAIST REACHES

1. With feet still parallel and knees slightly bent, pull over to the right, reaching both arms past your head to the right. Stretch for 8 counts.

Don't let your left shoulder pull forward. Feel the stretch up your left side.

2. Reach over to the left, stretching both arms past your head to the left. Stretch for 8 counts.

Don't let your right shoulder pull forward.

# 6 · SHOULDER STRETCH

1. Lace your fingers together behind your back. With knees bent, lean over and allow your arms to stretch forward over your head. Hold for 8 counts.

Your head should be relaxed, your back rounded.

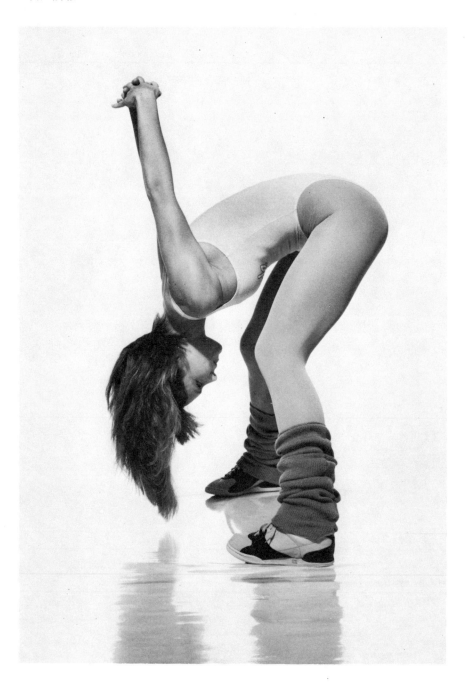

# 7 · HAMSTRING STRETCH

1. Keeping your knees slightly bent, clasp both ankles and stretch for 8 counts.

2. Slowly straighten your knees and gently press your chest toward your thighs. Stretch for 8 counts.

Repeat Steps 1 and 2 two more times.

BREATHE DEEPLY.

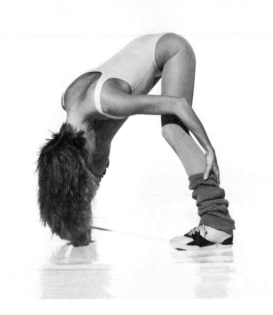

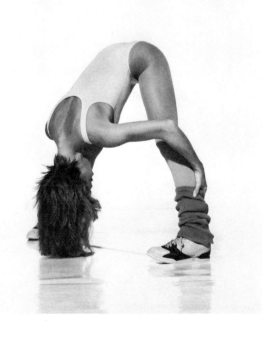

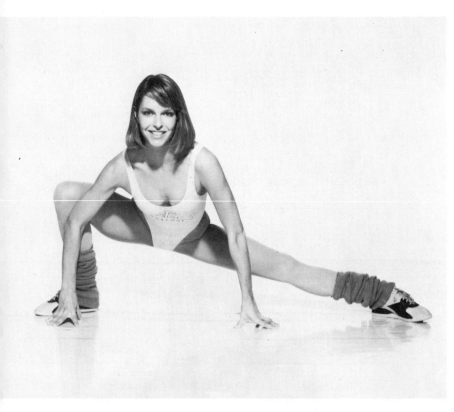

# $8 \cdot$ INNER THIGH STRETCH

1. Bend your knees. Place your hands on the floor in front of you. Slide your left leg out to the side as you bend your right knee, lowering your hips with arms inside your legs. Your right elbow presses your right knee open. Right heel is on the floor. Hold for 8 counts.

Feel the stretch in your inner thigh. Both feet are flat on the floor.

2. Shift your weight to the left leg and repeat to the other side for 8 counts. Your arms are still inside your legs, left elbow is pressing your left knee open.

Be sure not to let your knees roll inward.

3. Come center with legs straight and stretch down over your thighs.

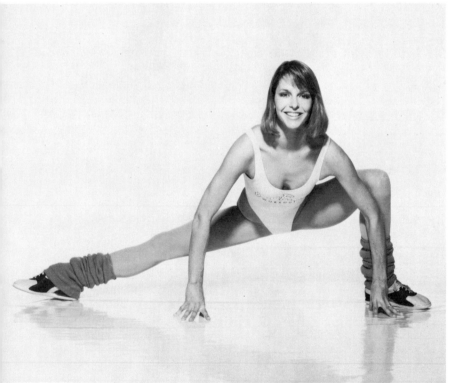

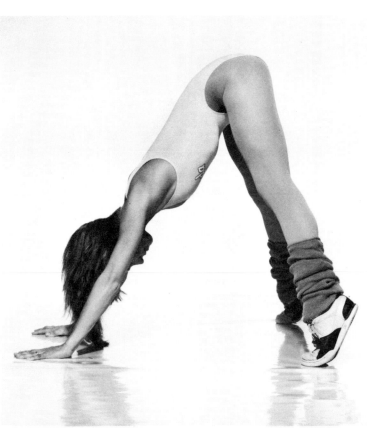

# 9 · TOE RAISES

1. Walk your hands out in front of you. With feet parallel, press up high on your toes . . .

2. then lower your heels. Press up and lower 30 times.

Keep your abdominals pulled in.

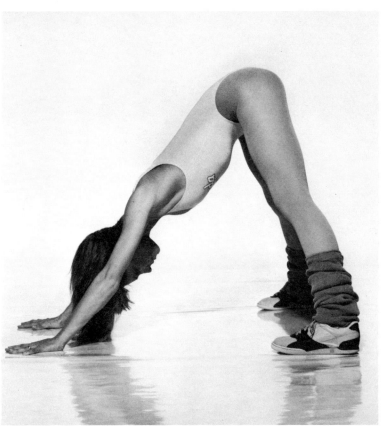

# 10 · TENDON STRETCH

1. Walk your feet together to about 4 inches apart. Lift your left heel and bend your left knee as you press your right heel to the floor for 4 counts.

2. Lift your right heel, bending the right knee, as you press your left heel toward the floor. Hold for 4 counts.

Right and left heel stretch is 1 set. Do 3 sets. Then press both heels toward the floor and hold for 4 counts.

Keep abdominals pulled in. Feel the stretch up the back of the legs.

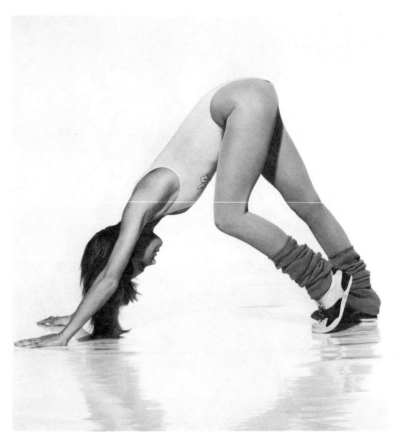

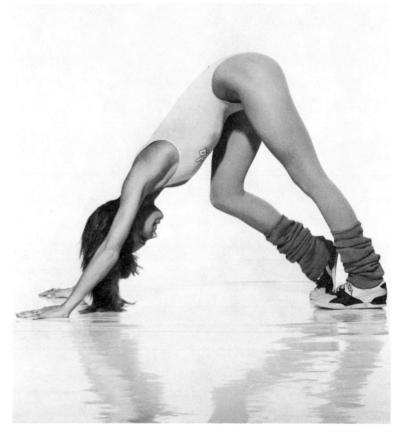

# 11 · PUSH-UPS

1. Lower yourself to the floor, both legs straight, and place your hands beneath your shoulders pointing front. Keeping your back flat . . .

2. inhale and bend your elbows, lowering your body as far as you can. Then exhale and straighten your arms again.

Do as many as you can without feeling strain in your lower back.

If these straight-legged push-ups are too difficult, do them with bent knees. (See page 111.)

*Do not arch your back.*

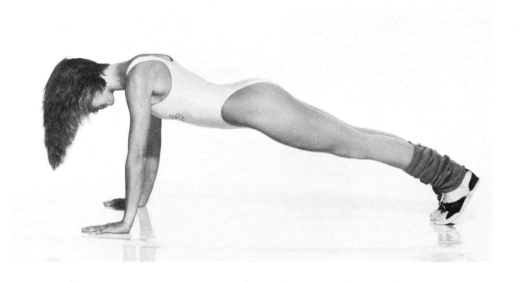

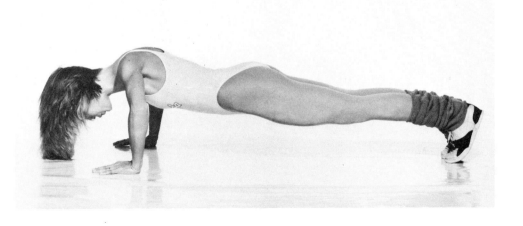

# 12 · TRICEPS PUSH-UPS

1. Sit on the floor with knees bent and hands and feet flat on the floor about a foot from your hips. Palms are shoulder-width apart, hands pointing forward.

2. Straighten your arms and press your body up. Then bend your elbows and lower your body until your buttocks just touch the floor.

Press up and lower 8 times.

EXHALE AS YOU PRESS UP.

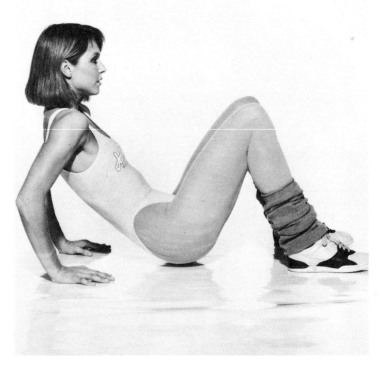

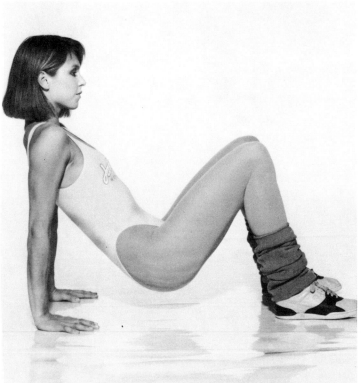

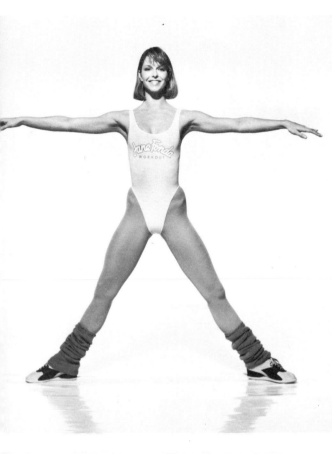

# 13 · PLIÉS

1. Stand with your legs *very* wide apart, feet slightly turned out, arms to the side at shoulder height.

2. Bend your knees so that your hips are almost on a level with your knees. Keep your knees pressed back.

3. Straighten your legs part way.

Steps 2 and 3 are 1 set. Do 16 sets.

Keep your pubic bone tucked upward to prevent your back from arching. Abdominals are pulled in, weight is slightly forward, knees are pressed back.

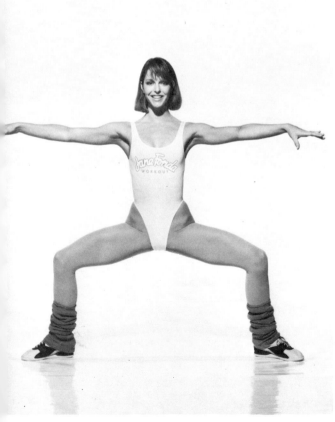

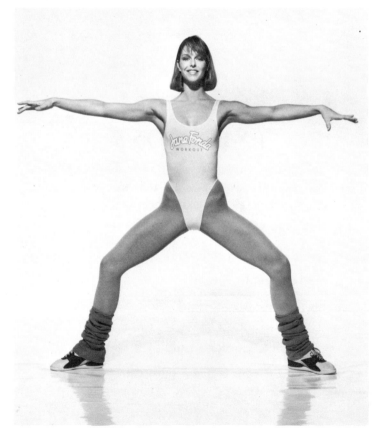

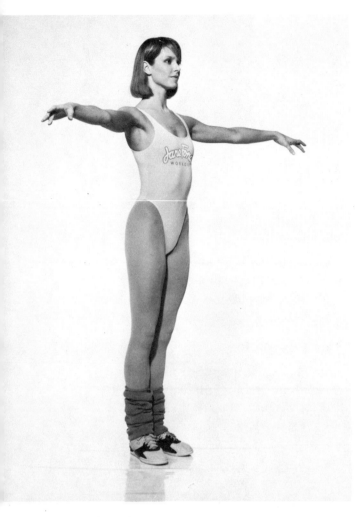
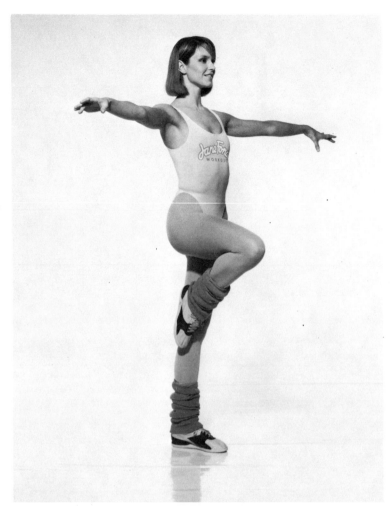

# 14 · LEG EXTENSIONS

1. Stand with your feet together, slightly turned out, arms out to the side at shoulder height. (Don't hunch up!)

2. Lift your right knee.

3. Extend your leg in front of you . . .

4. and bend it back again.

Steps 3 and 4 are done to 1 count.

5. Do 7 counts; on the 8th count lower your leg to rest for 1 count.

Repeat all 8 counts again with the same leg.

*(continued)*

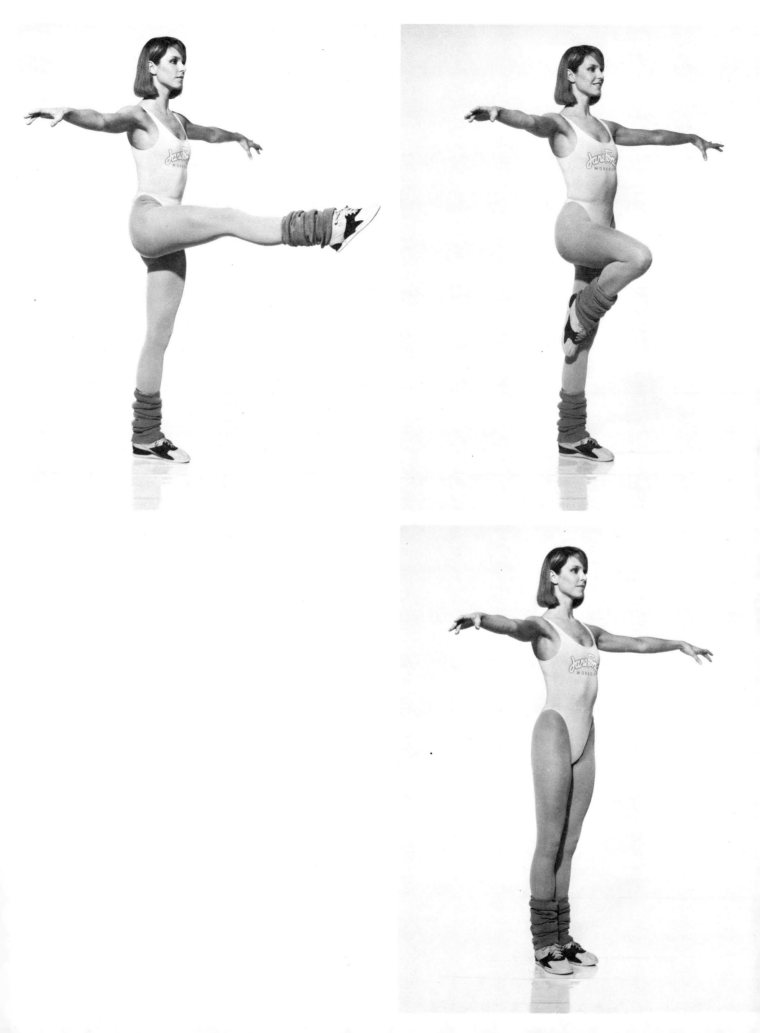

6. Repeat to the left side. Lift your left knee.

7. Extend your leg out in front of you . . .

8. and bend it back.

9. Repeat steps 7 and 8 for 7 counts; on the 8th count lower your leg to rest for 1 count.

Repeat all 8 counts again with same leg.

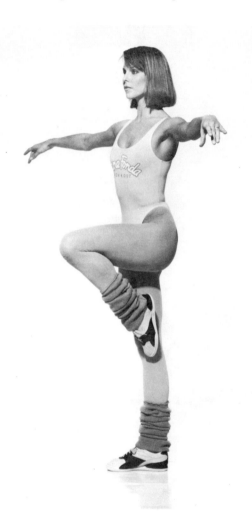

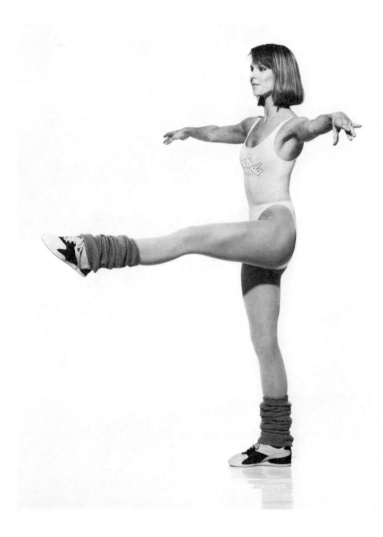

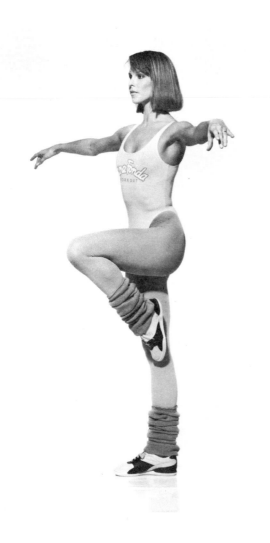
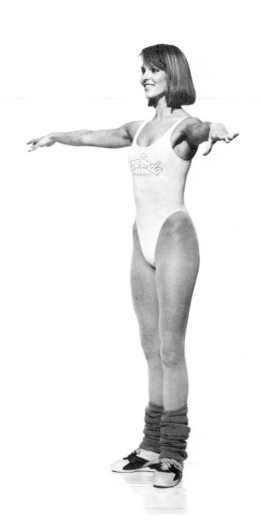

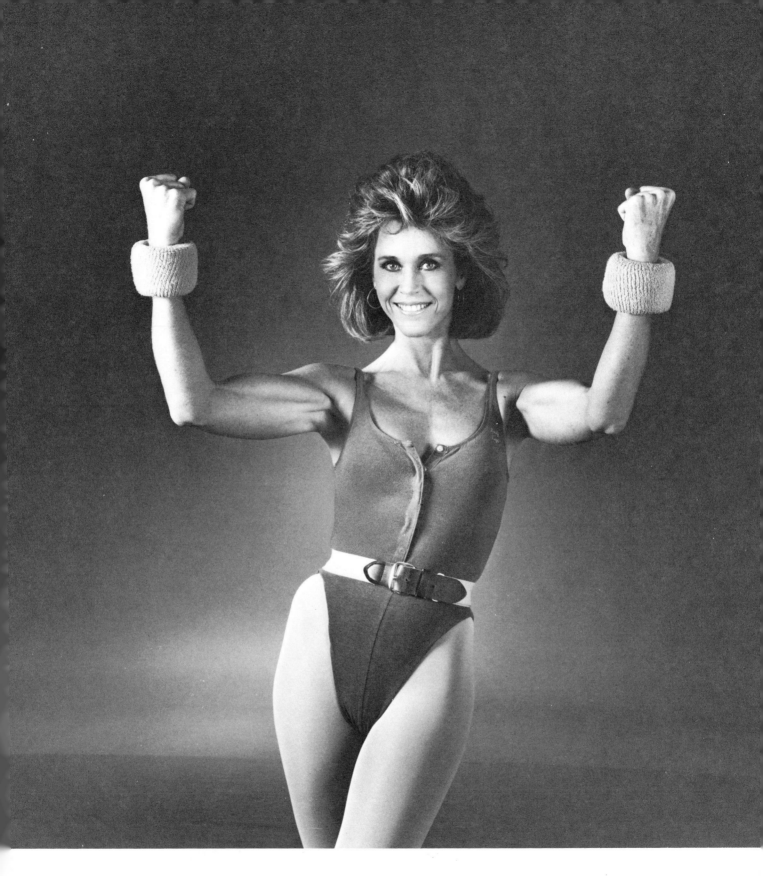

# Upper Body

*You may want to wear half-pound or one-pound wrist weights.*

# 1 · ARM CIRCLES

1. With knees bent and feet parallel (toes pointing forward) bring your arms to the side, shoulder level, and circle your arms *backward* with elbows slightly bent, hands flexed upward. Circle 32 times.

2. Continue circling backward with fists flexed downward, 32 times.

The circling motion is done with the entire arm moving from the shoulder; as the arms move backward think of pressing your shoulder blades together. Don't let the shoulders hunch up. Knees remain bent.

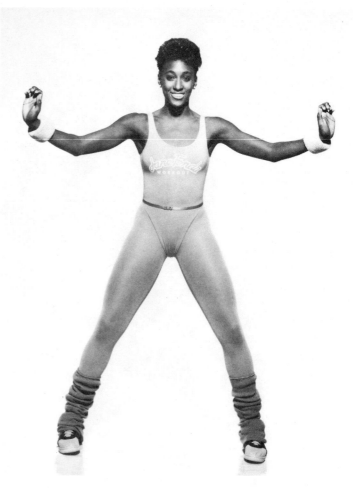

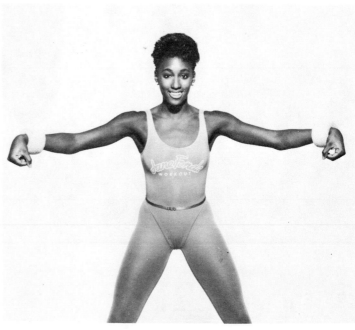

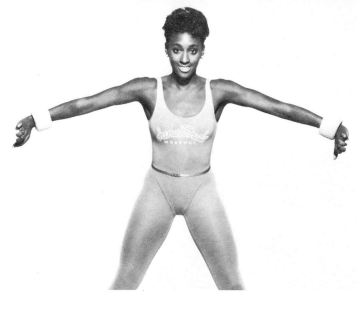

# 2 · ELBOW EXTENSIONS

1. Raise your arms to shoulder height and rotate them forward from the shoulders as far as possible. The inside of your wrists should be facing upward.

2. Bring your lower arms in toward your body . . .

3. then extend them down and out to shoulder height with the inside of the wrists facing upward. Feel you are resisting a pressure as you extend your arms.

Steps 2 and 3 are done to 1 count. Repeat for a total of 32 counts.

Keep your elbows at shoulder height. Don't let your shoulders hunch up. Think of making a half circle with your lower arms.

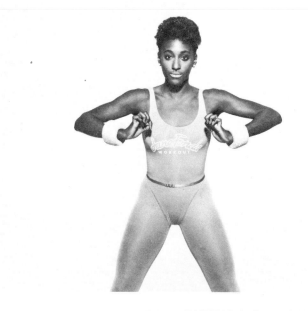

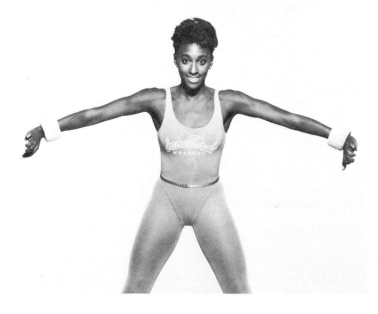

# 3 · SHOULDER TWISTS

1. Extend your arms to the side at shoulder height, palms up.

2. Rotate your arms forward from the shoulders until your palms are facing up again . . .

3. then rotate the arms back again to starting position.

These 2 rotations are 1 set. Do 16 sets.

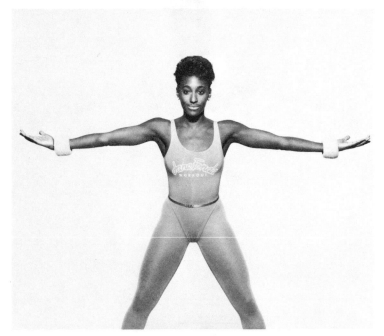

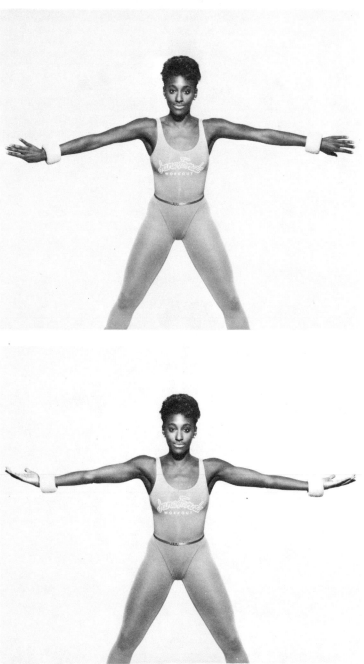

# 4 · BICEPS CURLS

1. Bring your clenched fists in toward
   your shoulders . . .

2. and extend them out again.

Steps 1 and 2 are done to 1 count. Do 16
counts.

Keep your chest lifted. Resist the inward
movement and tighten the biceps muscles.

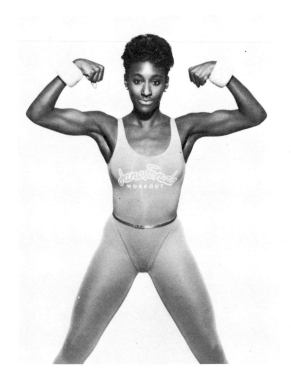

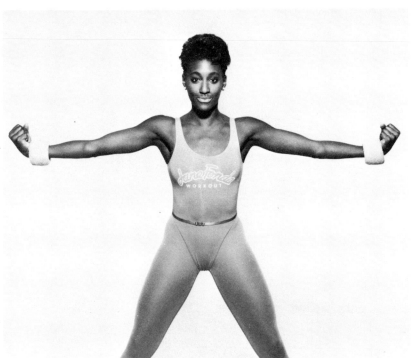

# 5 · PECTORAL PRESSES

1. Keeping both knees slightly bent, bend your elbows at right angles . . .

2. then press your elbows together, resisting the motion.

3. Open them out again.

Press and open to 1 count. Do 24 counts.

As you press inward, imagine you are pressing a big beach ball . . . feel the resistance.

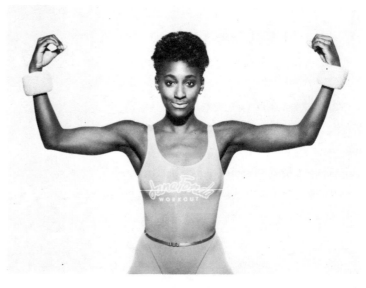

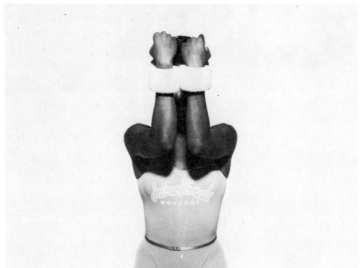

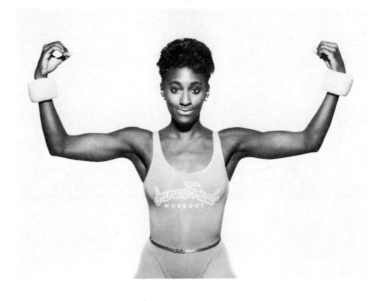

# 6 · TRICEPS EXTENSIONS

1. Keeping your knees bent, bend forward from the hips with a flat back. Elbows are bent up behind you, fists held at the sides of your breasts.

2. Extend your arms behind you as high as you can with inside of wrists facing downward.

3. Bend arms in again to starting position.

Steps 2 and 3 are done to 1 count. Repeat for 15 counts.

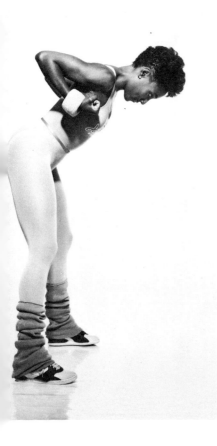
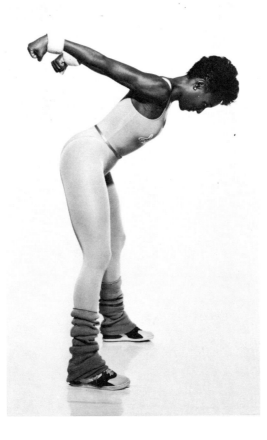
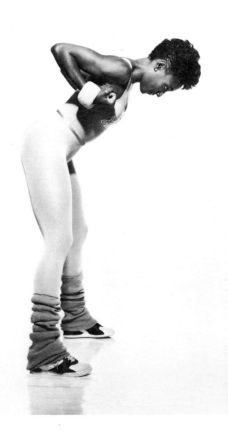

# 7 · DELTOID PRESSES

1. Extend your arms behind your back with hands open, palms facing upward . . .

2. and press them upward 16 times (lowering them a little between each press).

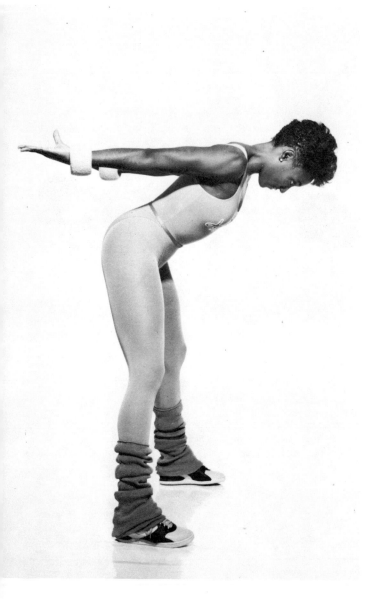
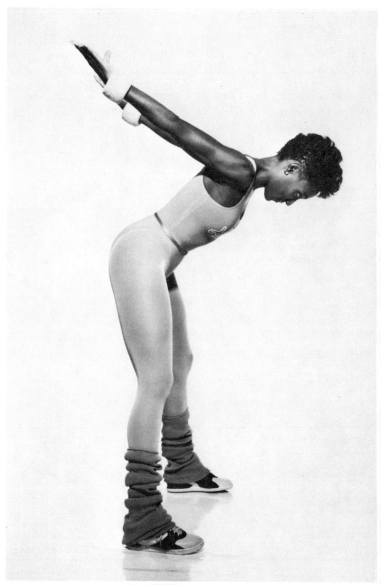

# 8 · SIDE ARM-LIFTS

1. Bring your bent arms down in front of you . . .

2. then lift them out to the side with elbows still slightly bent.

Steps 1 and 2 are done to 1 count. Repeat for a total of 16 counts.

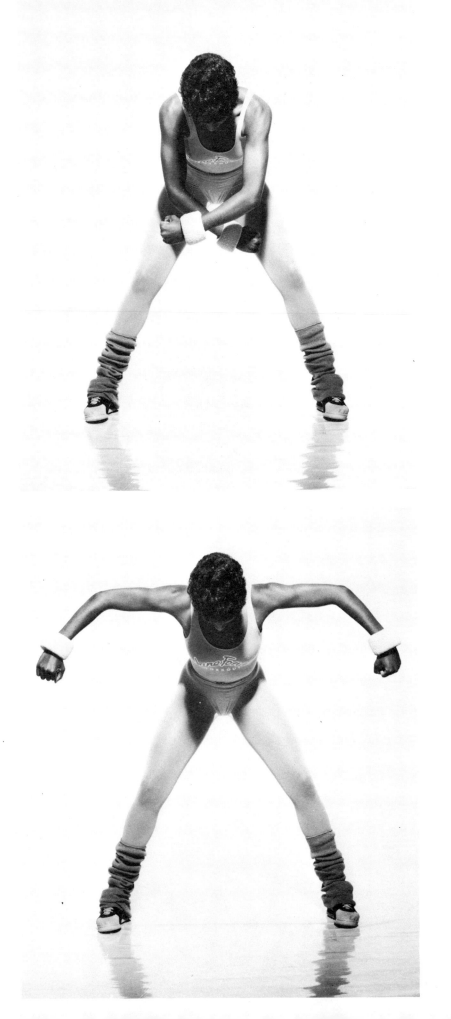

# 9 · SHOULDER STRETCH

1. Standing upright again, bend your right arm behind your head and press your right elbow downward with your left hand. Hold for 4 long counts.

2. Repeat to the left. Bend your left arm behind your head and press your left elbow downward with your right hand. Hold for 4 long counts.

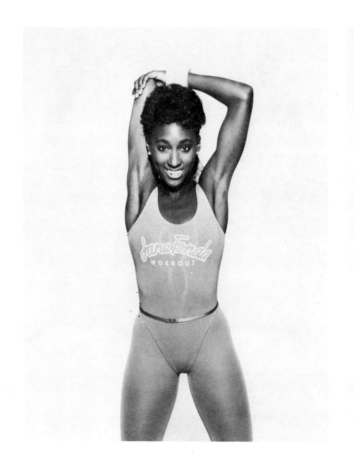
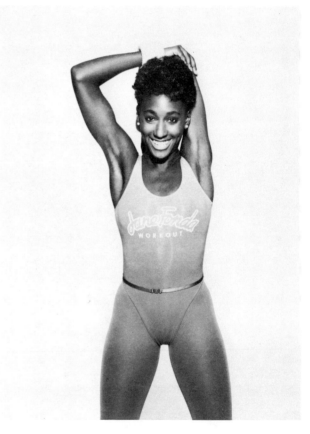

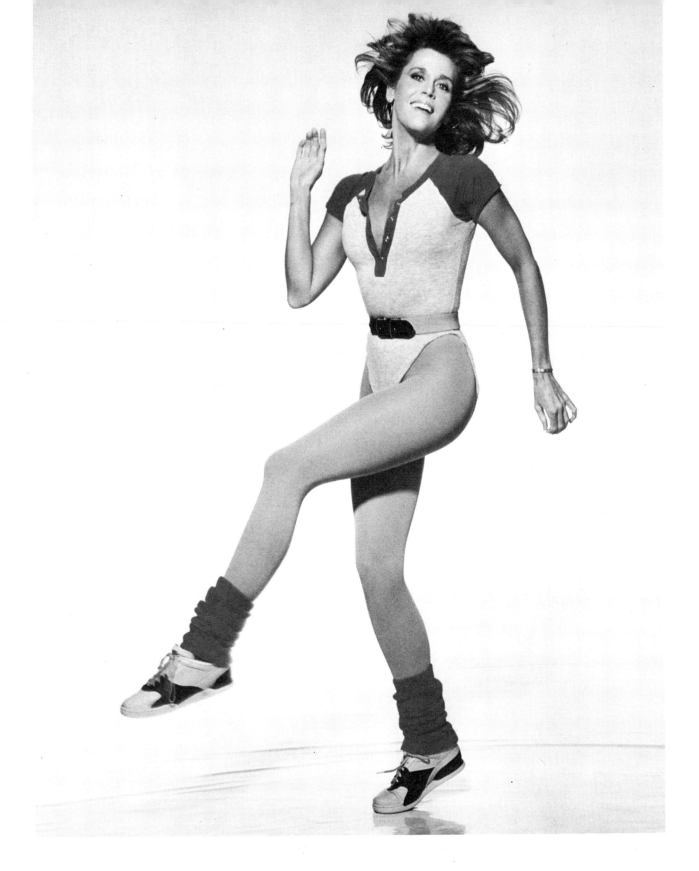

# Aerobics

# HOW TO DO IT

Be sure you are wearing good, supportive aerobic shoes.

Put on music that makes you want to move and dance. That's what will motivate you. Your goal is to do 30 to 40 minutes of nonstop aerobic movement.

Start with 5 minutes of small steps in place, lifting your feet only slightly, to gradually raise your pulse rate.

Follow this with 5 minutes of small jogging steps in place. Then begin the more vigorous steps such as skipping, step-kicks, jumping jacks, prancing, can-can kicks, etc. The more you work with your arms overhead, the more you will increase your pulse rate.

To be sure that you are burning your stored fat, you should be doing steps that will allow you to carry on a conversation without becoming excessively breathless yet keep your pulse rate within its training zone. At the 15-minute mark, stop and take your pulse. If you are not at your training level push yourself harder by taking larger steps, lifting your knees and legs higher, and doing more of the steps with your arms overhead. (See page 78 for instructions on how to determine your proper training zone.) To increase your aerobic output try wearing half-pound to one-pound wrist weights while doing aerobics. Don't go above one pound and do not wear ankle weights—they will put too much strain on your joints.

The more you vary your steps, the more you will dissipate the stress to your joints and shins. It will also help lessen the impact if you move about over an area at least 3 to 4 feet square as you dance/jog. The more room you have to move about in, the better.

Most important:

---

- Breathe deeply throughout.
- Land on the balls of your feet and allow your heels to touch down.
- Pull up tall. Don't slouch.
- Land with bent knees.
- Don't stop abruptly. Give your heart rate a chance to slow down gradually.

---

Instead of doing 30 to 40 minutes of aerobic dancing to music, you can take a brisk 40- to 50-minute walk, or jog, ride a stationary bike, or do any other aerobic activity. Just be sure to get your cardiovascular work done *at least* 3 to 4 times a week.

# Aerobic Cool-down

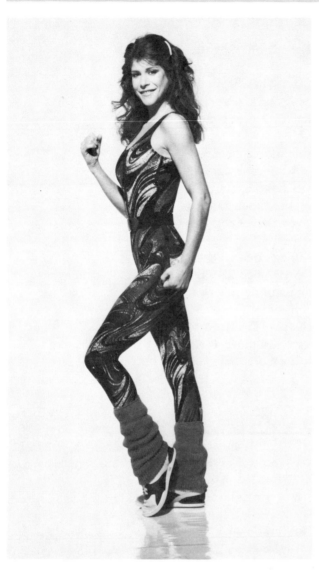 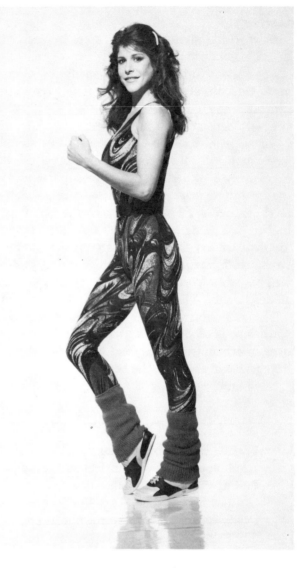

1. For several minutes take prancing steps without jumping . . .

2. . . . while your heart rate begins to slow down and you catch your breath.

3. Then with your legs wide apart, hands on your knees, bend your knees . . .

4. and gently straighten them. Bend and straighten 8 times.

5. Walk your hands on the floor way out in front of you and press your right heel into the floor . . .

6. then press the left heel into the floor. Pressing right and left is 1 set. Do 8 sets.

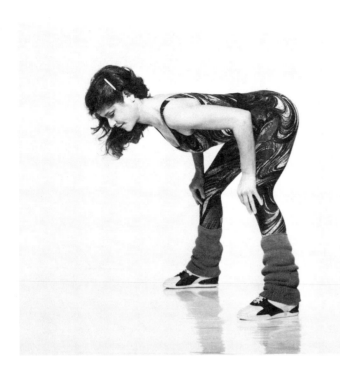 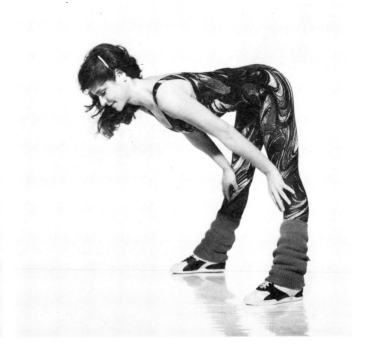

Abdominals are pulled in, hips are stretching up toward the ceiling, pubic bone is curling toward your navel.

(continued)

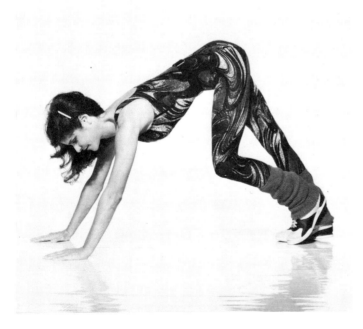 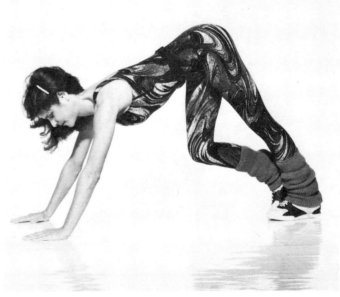

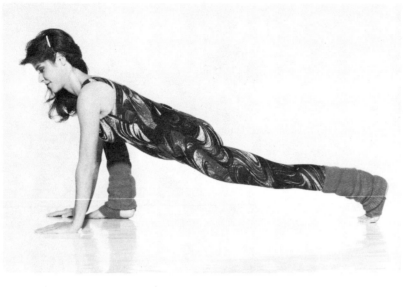

7. Bring right foot flat on the floor in front of you with right knee bent, left leg extended out behind you. Hands are on the floor on either side of your bent leg, hips pressing forward. Press hips forward for 8 counts.

8. Shift your weight back, straightening your front leg, and flex your front foot. Stretch your chest down over your thigh and stretch your back heel toward the floor. Hold the stretch for 8 counts. Don't let your right hip ride out to the side. Keep it aligned with your left hip.

9. Bend your right knee again and stretch your hips forward.

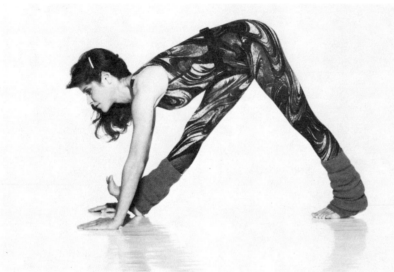

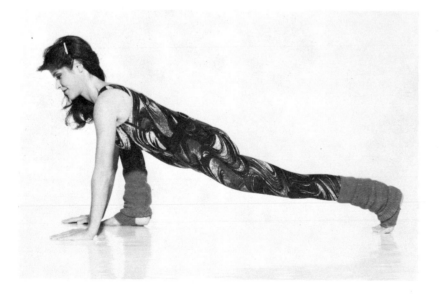

10. Bend your back (left) leg. Slide that knee as far as you can behind you. Reach around with the *opposite* hand (right), clasp your left foot, and press it gently toward your buttocks. Hold for 8 counts. Keep your hips pressed forward.

11. Release that foot, extend both legs behind you . . .

12. and bring your left leg in front of you, foot flat on the floor, leaving your right leg extended behind. Press hips forward for 8 counts.

*(continued)*

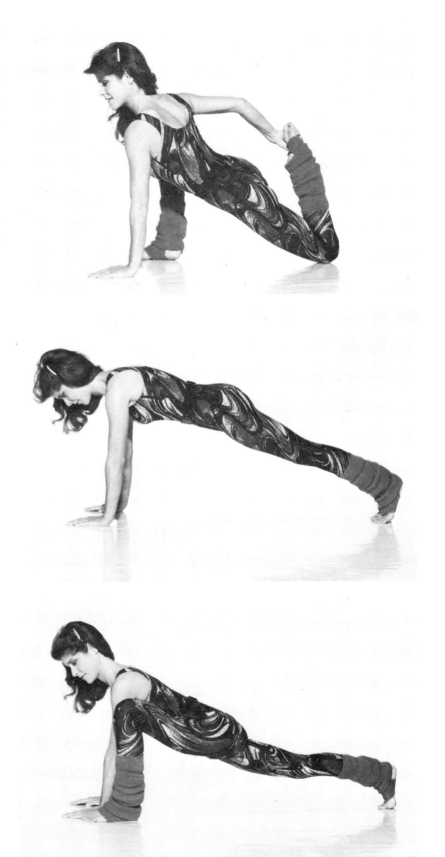

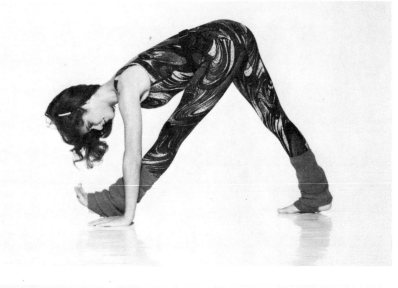

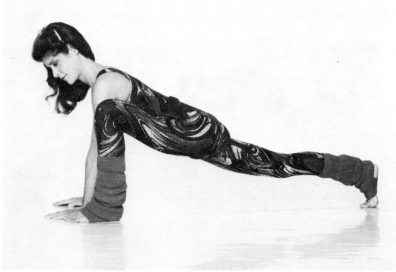

13. Shift your weight back, straightening your front leg, and flex your front foot. Stretch your chest down over your thigh and stretch your back heel toward the floor. Hold for 8 counts. Don't let your left hip ride out to the side. Keep it aligned with your right hip.

14. Bend your left knee again and stretch your hips forward.

15. Bend your right leg. Slide that knee as far as you can behind you. Reach around with the *opposite* hand (left), clasp your right foot, and press it gently toward your buttocks. Hold for 8 counts. Keep your hips pressed forward.

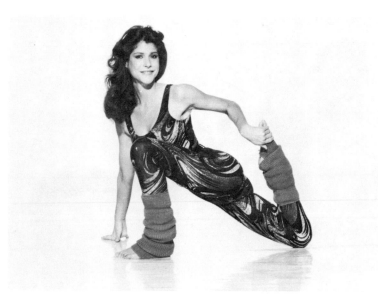

16. Release that foot and stand, bringing both feet together with knees bent, torso stretching down over your thighs, hands behind your ankles.

17. Keeping your torso against your thighs, straighten your legs.

18. Bend knees again . . .

*(continued)*

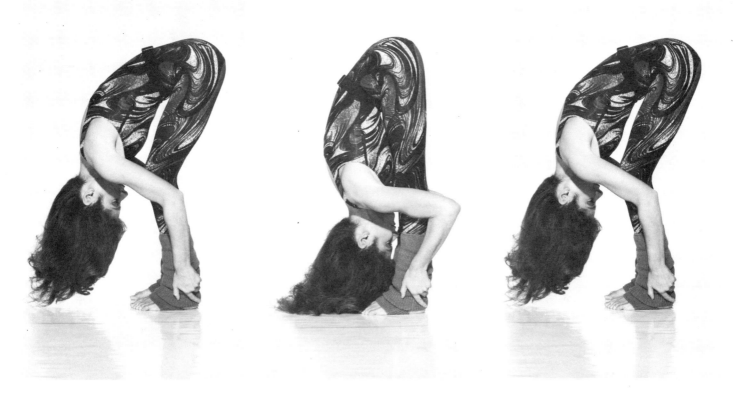

19. and slowly roll up, one vertebra at a time . . .

20. to a standing position.

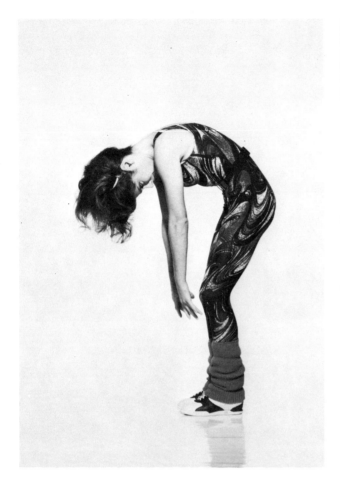 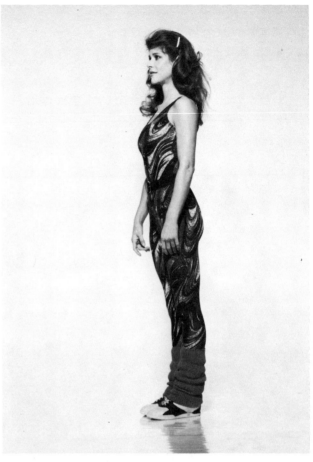

*Get yourself a towel, folded blanket, or mat and we'll go on to floor work.*

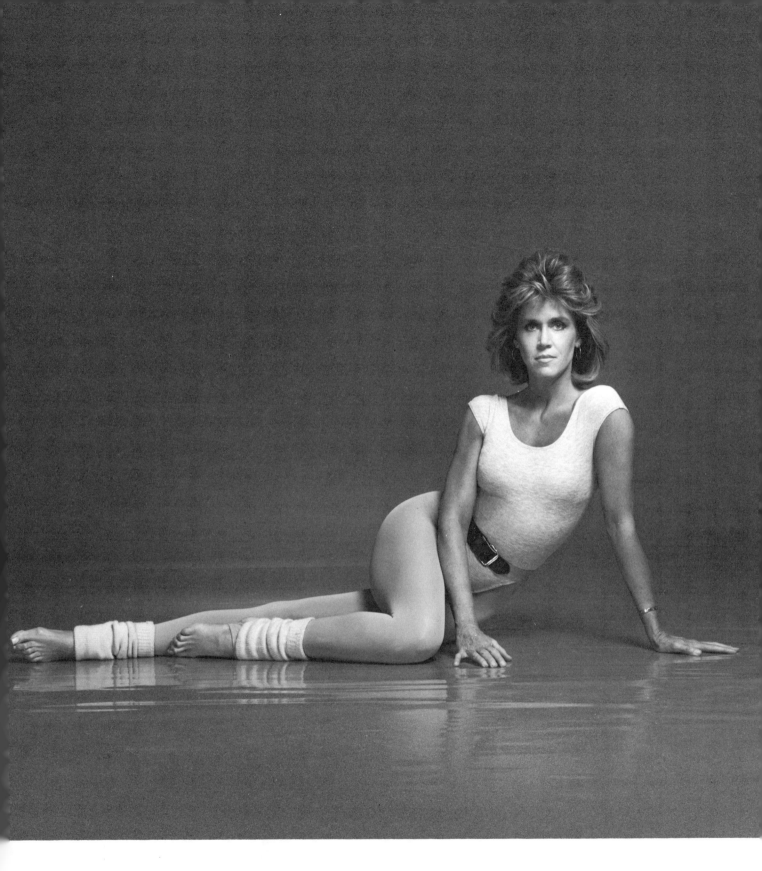

# Floor Stretch

*You should remove your shoes now. These stretches should be done on a mat or blanket to cushion your hips and back and keep dust out of your nose and hair.*

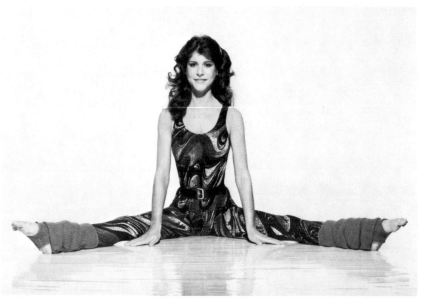

# 1 · FLOOR STRETCH

1. Sitting on the floor, open your legs as wide as you can without straining. Point your toes.

2. Pull over to the right side. Your left arm is reaching directly over your head to the right. Press your left shoulder back. Hold for 16 counts, stretching and lengthening the left side. Don't bounce.

3. Turn and face your right leg, hands on either side of it. Reach out over that leg with your torso for 8 counts. Press your left hip into the floor.

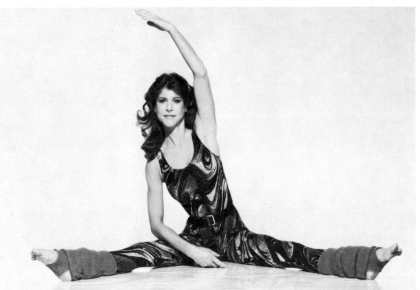

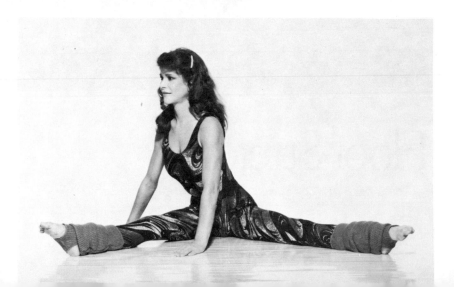

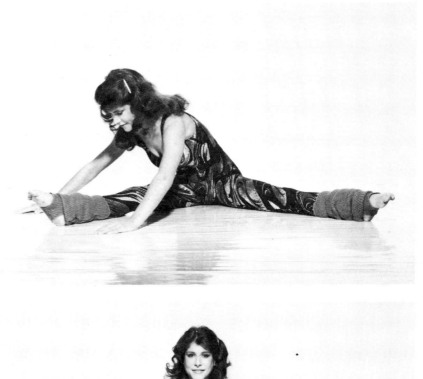

4. Round your back and pull down over your right leg. Stretch and breathe for 8 counts.

5. Roll torso back up to center position, then . . .

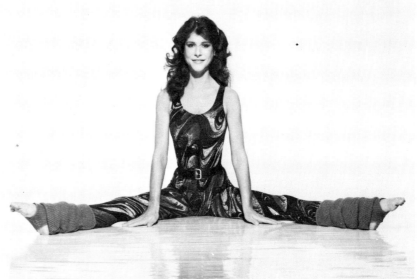

6. repeat to the left, pulling over to the side with your right arm reaching directly overhead. Press your right shoulder back. Hold for 16 counts, stretching and lengthening the right side. Don't bounce.

*(continued)*

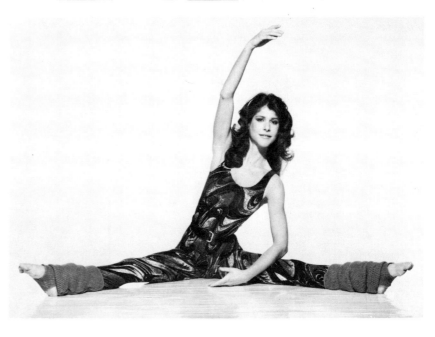

7. Turn and face your left leg. Reach out over that leg with your torso for 8 counts. Press your right hip into the floor.

8. Round your back and pull down over your left leg. Stretch and breathe for 8 counts.

9. With your hands on the floor in front of you, "walk" yourself to the center, flex your feet, and stretch out over the floor, lengthening your spine for 16 counts.

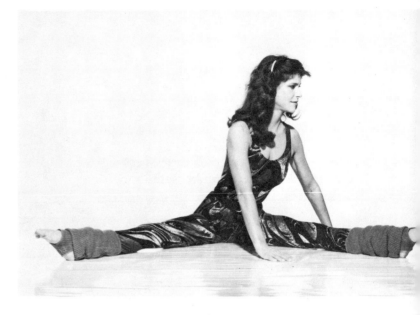

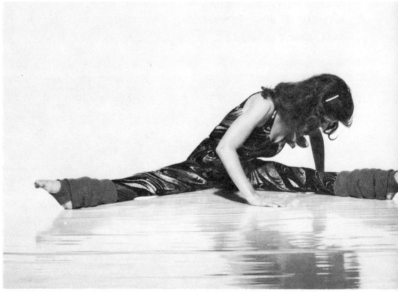

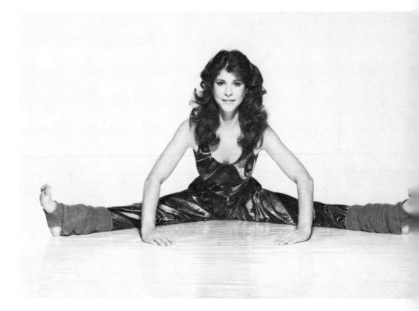

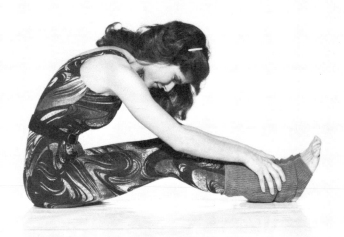

# 2 · HAMSTRING STRETCH

1. Bring your legs together in front of you with feet flexed and knees slightly bent. Round your head and torso down over your legs and hold for 12 counts. Don't hold your breath.

2. Bend your knees more, pull in your abdominals, and roll up to a sitting position.

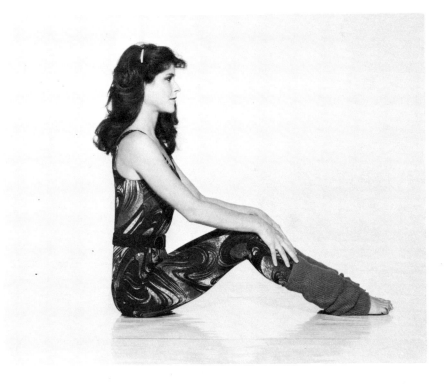

*Now roll onto your back and go right into the abdominal work.*

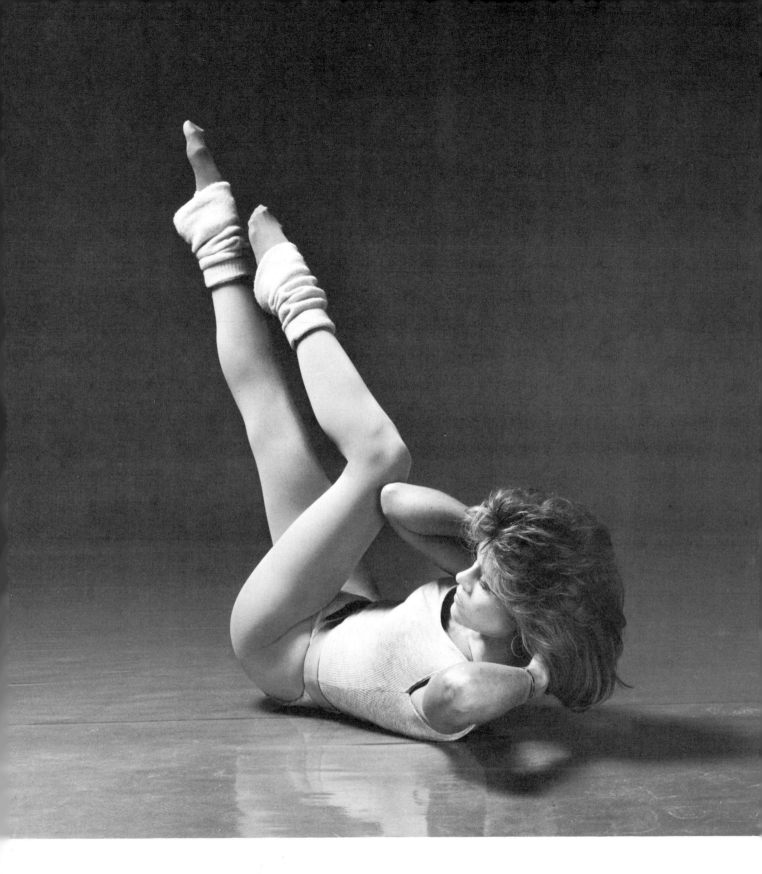

# Abdominals

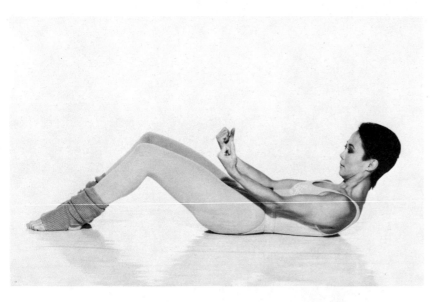

# 1 · KNEE-LIFTS

1. Roll down onto your back with knees bent, feet hip-distance apart. Fists in front of thighs, tuck chin to chest . . .

2. and lift your bent right knee and your arms to your chest as you sit up.

3. Put your right foot down again and extend your arms in front of thighs as you release back part way.

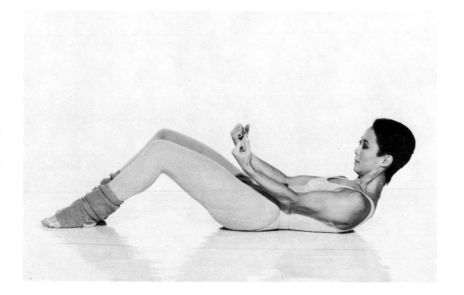

4. Then bring your left knee and your arms to your chest as you sit up.

5. Replace your left foot and extend your arms as you release back part way.

Right and left knee-lifts are 1 set. Do 8 sets.

Exhale as you sit up. Inhale as you release.

6. Repeat the basic movement of step 2, but as you sit up cross your left elbow over to your right knee.

*(continued)*

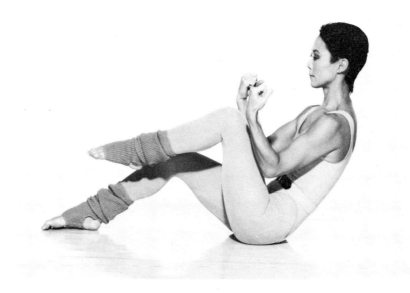

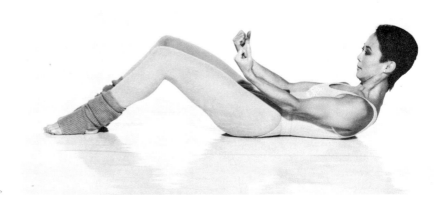

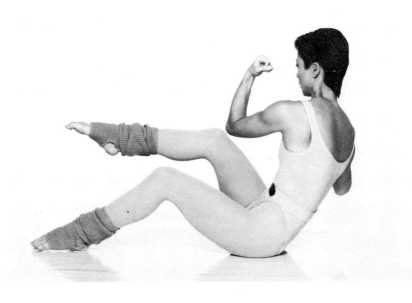

7. Put your right foot down again and extend your arms in front of thighs as you release back part way.

8. Bring your right elbow over to your left knee as you sit up.

9. Replace your left foot and extend your arms as you release back part way.

Steps 6, 7, 8, 9 are 1 set. Do 8 sets.

EXHALE AS YOU SIT UP; INHALE AS YOU RELEASE.

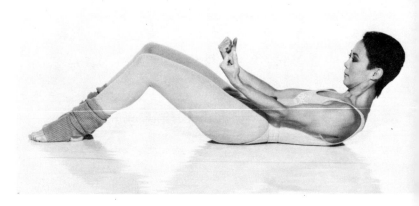

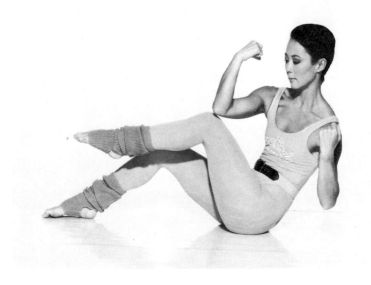

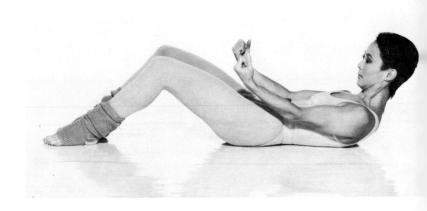

# 2 · LEG EXTENSION SIT-UPS

1. Lying flat on your back, reach straight up with your right leg and extend left leg out parallel to the floor, toes pointed. With hands behind your head, lift your upper body toward your right leg . . .

2. and lower part way. Lift and lower 8 times.

3. Reach straight up with your left leg, your right leg stretched parallel to the floor. Lift your upper body toward your left leg . . .

4. and lower part way. Lift and lower 8 times.

*(continued)*

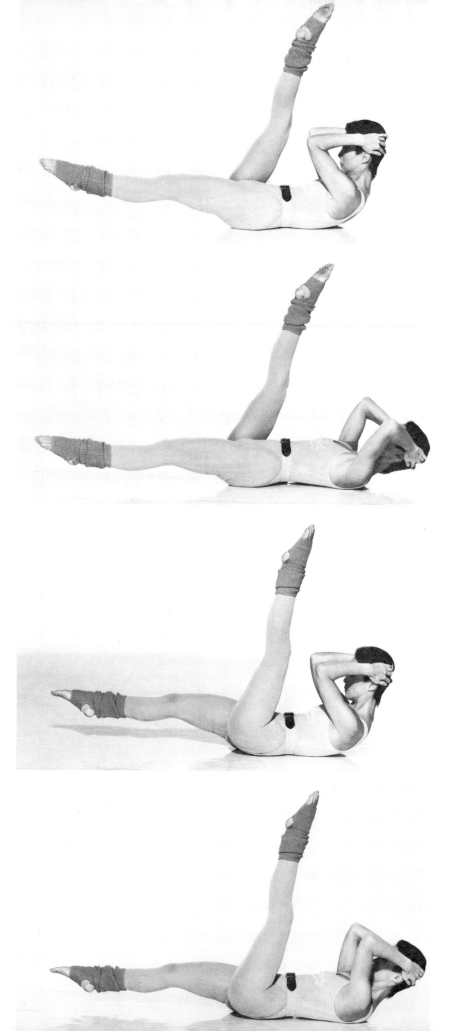

5. Then do 8 sit-ups with both legs up, releasing part way between each sit-up.

EXHALE AS YOU COME UP. INHALE AS YOU RELEASE.

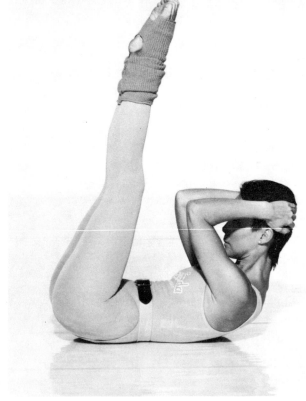

If you feel any strain in your lower back, place your hands beneath your hips as you do these sit-ups.

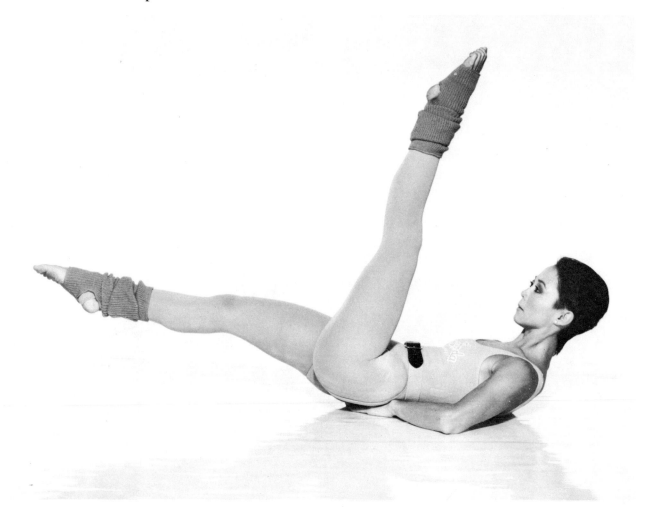

# 3 · CRUNCHES

1. Bend your legs slightly, and cross your ankles. Hands are behind your head with elbows pointing forward.

2. Reach up toward your knees with your upper body, then release back slightly.

Reach and release 32 times.

EXHALE AS YOU REACH; INHALE AS YOU RELEASE.

The movement is very small. Try to keep your shoulder blades off the floor, even when you release. Use your abdominals to raise your upper body, not your arms.

Without breaking rhythm go right on to . . .

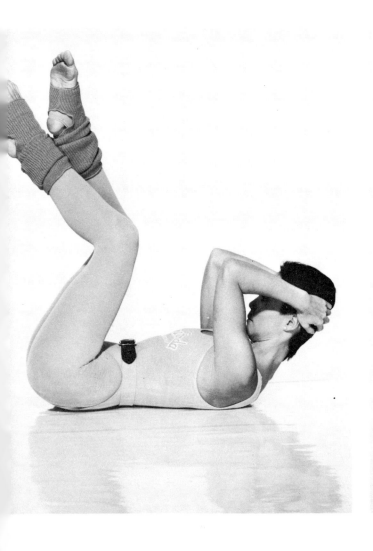 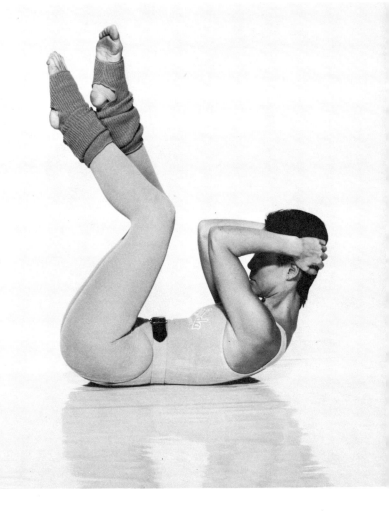

# 4 · CROSSOVERS

1. Reach your right elbow across to the outside of your left knee . . .

2. then, trying not to let the shoulders release back very much, reach your left elbow to the outside of your right knee.

Reaching right and left is 1 set. Do 24 sets.

These movements work the oblique muscles along the side of the waist.

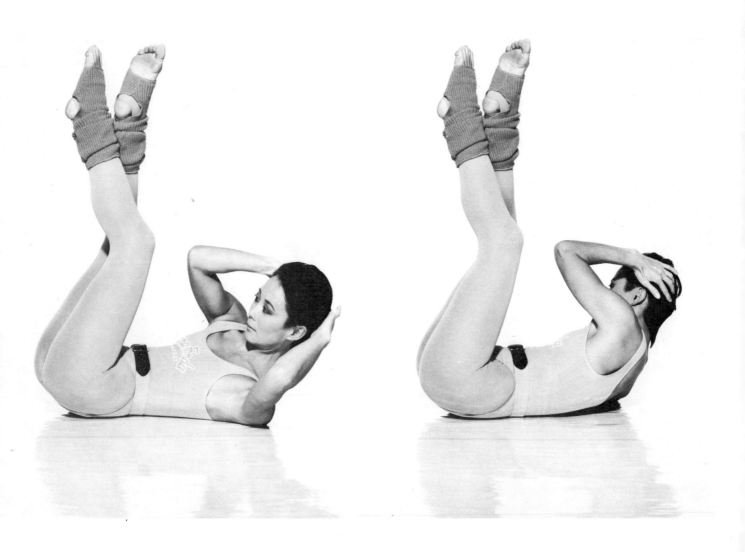

# 5 · BICYCLES

1. With hands behind head, extend the right leg straight out, toes pointed. Bend your left knee to your chest, reaching your right elbow over to touch the outside of your left knee.

2. Switch sides, extending the left leg out with toes pointed. Bend your right knee in and touch the left elbow to the right knee.

Steps 1 and 2 are 1 set. Do 4 sets slowly, 8 sets double time.

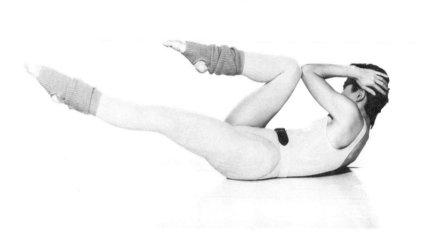

Repeat steps 1 and 2 with feet flexed.

Do 4 sets slowly, 8 sets double time.

And again, steps 1 and 2:
4 sets slowly with toes pointed,
8 sets double time.
4 sets slowly with feet flexed,
8 sets double time.

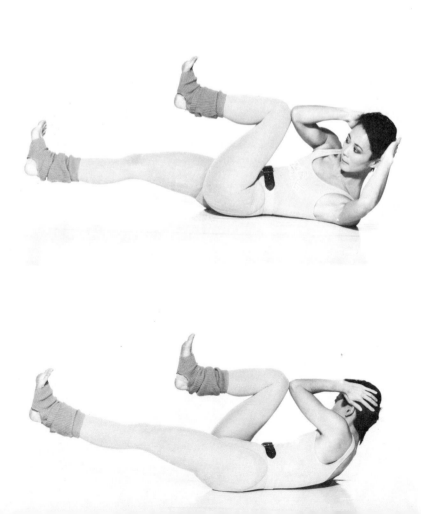

# 6 · SIT-UPS

1. Hands behind your head, elbows out to the side. Lift your head and upper body off the floor as high as you can in 2 counts . . .

2. then take 2 counts to lower part way, but do not touch the floor.

Lift and lower 4 times.

Repeat faster (using single counts) 8 times.

Then repeat slowly (using 2 counts to lift, 2 counts to lower) 4 times.

And faster (using single counts) 8 times.

EXHALE AS YOU LIFT, INHALE AS YOU LOWER.

All the lifting is done with the abdominals, not the arms. Don't put pressure on your neck with your hands.

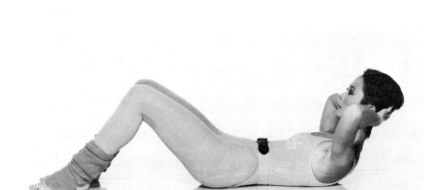

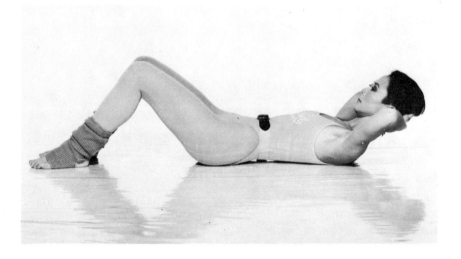

# 7 · MORNING STAR

Extend your left leg straight out on the floor. Bend your right knee, cross it over the left, and press it down toward the floor on the left side with your left hand. Be sure to curl your pubic bone up toward your navel. Your right arm is extended straight out to the side from the shoulder. Try to press your right shoulder to the floor. Hold for 8 counts.

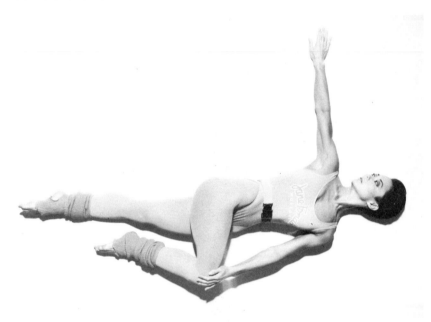

Repeat to the left: your right leg is extended straight out on the floor. Bend your left knee, cross it over the right, and press it down toward the floor on the right side with your right hand. Again, tuck the pubic bone up toward your navel. Your left arm is extended straight out to the side from the shoulder. Press your left shoulder to the floor. Hold for 8 counts.

This exercise stretches the abdominals, the hips, and the shoulder, and it decompresses the spine.

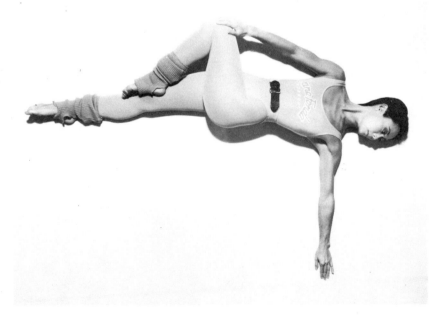

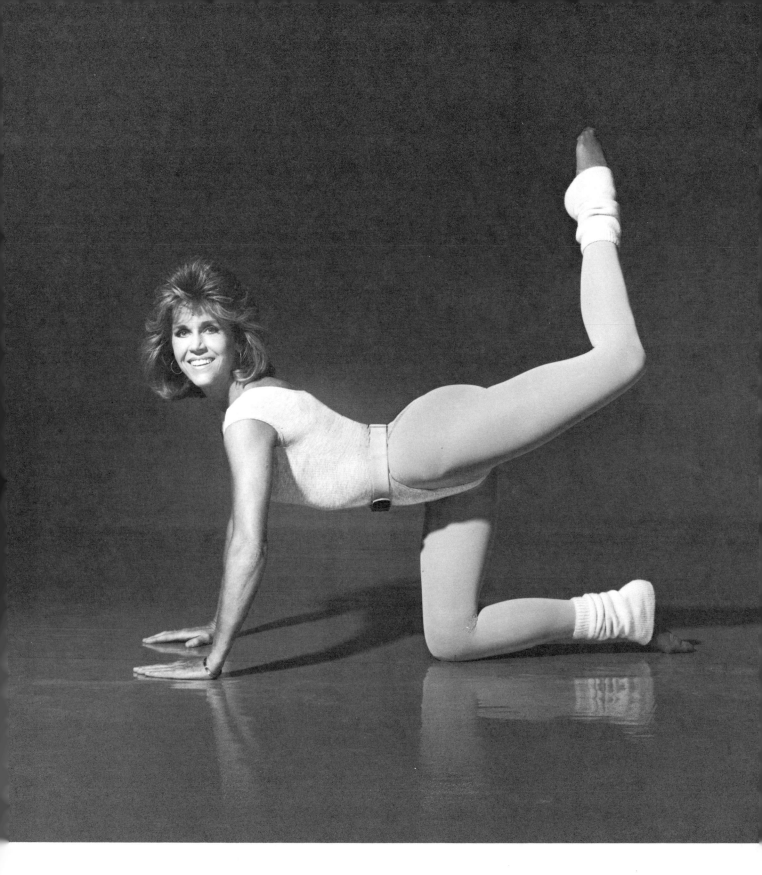

# Legs and Hips

*Go through all the leg and hip exercises using your right leg, as illustrated. When you finish the series, repeat each exercise using the left leg.*

*You may want to wear ankle weights.*

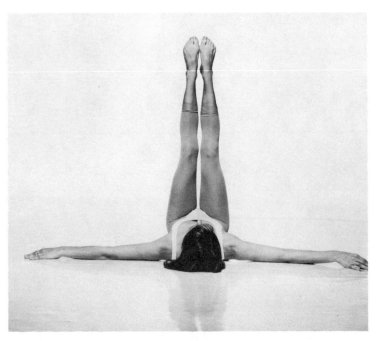

# 1 · INNER THIGHS

1. Lie on your back, arms out to the side, legs straight up in the air, toes pointed.

2. Open your legs wide . . .

3. and flex your feet as you bring your legs together and cross one over the other.

Steps 2 and 3 are 1 set. Do 24 sets, alternating the leg that closes in front.

Resist the closing of the legs so that you really work that inner thigh muscle.

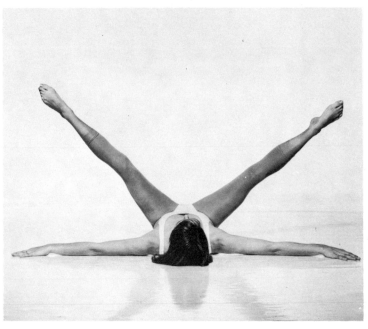

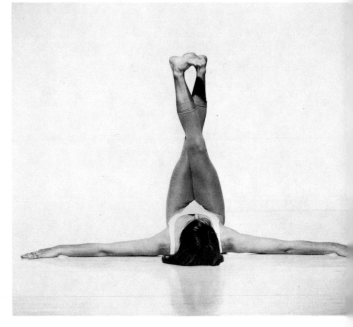

# 2 · PARALLEL LEG LIFTS

1. Lie on your left side, up on your elbow with palms flat on the floor. Extend both legs straight out on a line with your torso.

2. Point your toes and slowly lift your right leg as high as you can with your right hip pressing forward.

3. Slowly lower your leg part way. Don't let it touch your bottom leg.

Lift and lower 24 times.

*Be sure your top hip is pressing forward; don't rock back. Keep leg stretched out long as you lift it. Don't sink into your shoulder; lengthen the torso.*

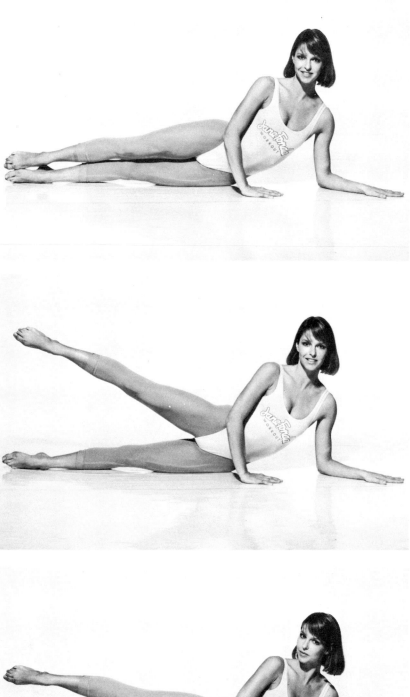

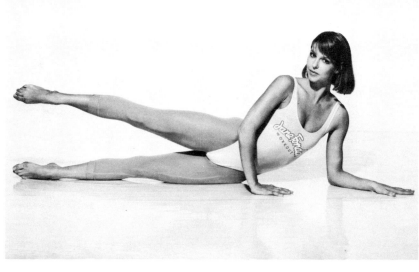

# 3 · LEG LIFTS

1. Bend your bottom knee and bring it out in front of you. Flex your right foot.

2. In a faster tempo lift your right leg . . .

3. and lower it part way.

Lift and lower 24 times.

Keep your weight forward on the hand in front of you.

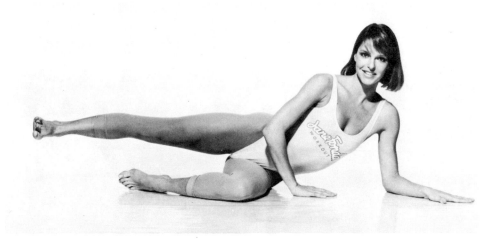

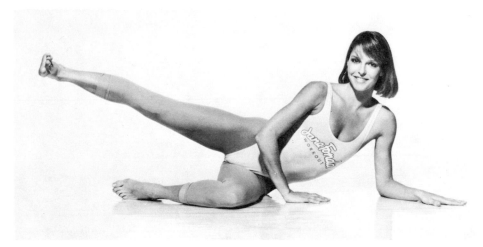

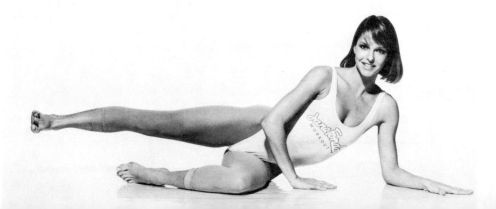

# 4 · FORWARD LEG EXTENSIONS

1. With bottom leg still bent, lift your bent right leg . . .

2. and extend it out from your body at a right angle. The right foot is flexed hard. (If you need to, hold on to that right leg to give it support.)

3. Bend your right knee again, without letting the right thigh move.

Straighten and bend 16 times.

Think of lengthening the leg, pushing out from the heel, as you straighten it. This will pull your top (right) hip forward.

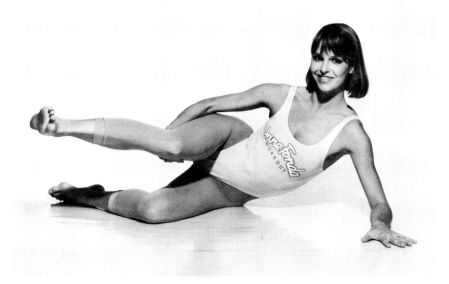

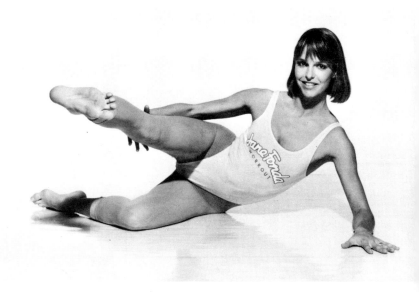

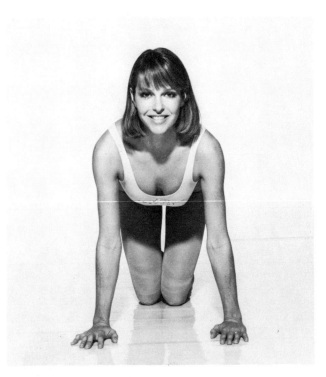

# 5 · ROVER'S REVENGE

1. On your hands and knees with weight evenly distributed, your stomach pulled in, pubic bone curled toward your navel . . .

2. lift your bent right knee out to the side to hip height . . .

3. then lower your knee almost to the floor.

Lift and lower 24 times.

4. Then do 16 small lifts from a raised position . . .

5. lowering the knee just a few inches between lifts.

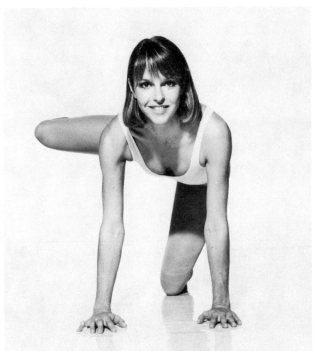

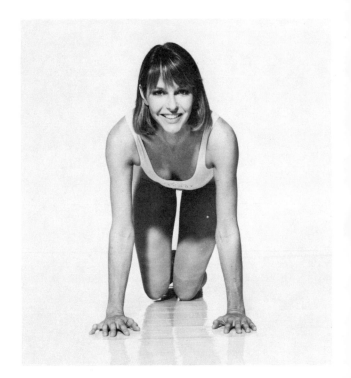

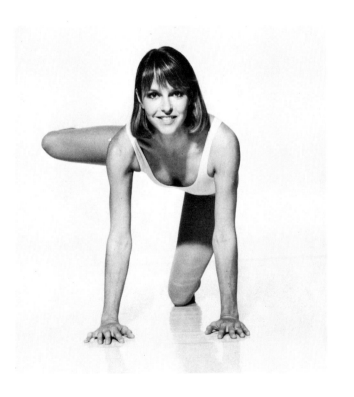
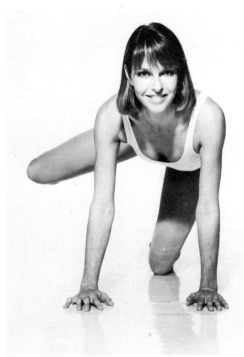

# 6 · BENT LEG LIFTS

1. Come down onto your elbows, head down, and with pointed toes and buttocks squeezed tight . . .

2. Lift your bent right leg behind you as high as you can without straightening it . . .

3. and lower your leg again, knee almost to the floor.

Lift and lower 24 times.

4. Then do 24 small lifts from a raised position with buttocks squeezed tight . . .

5. lowering just a few inches between lifts. (It's a very small, intense movement.)

Exhale as you lift. Inhale as you lower.

Don't let your back arch as you lift your leg. Keep your buttocks squeezed tight and your pubic bone tucked toward your navel. Your leg should lift against the resistance of your contracted buttock muscles.

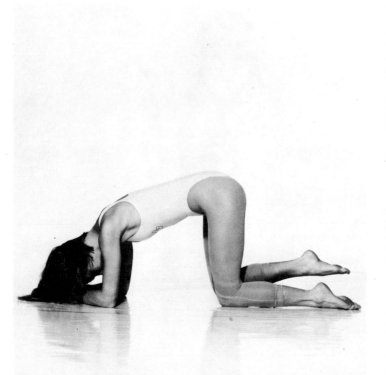
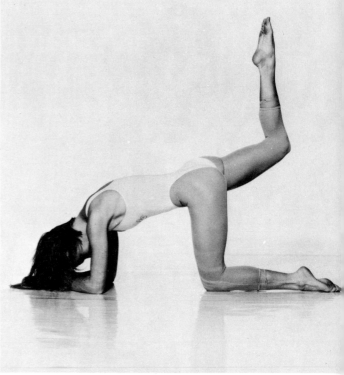

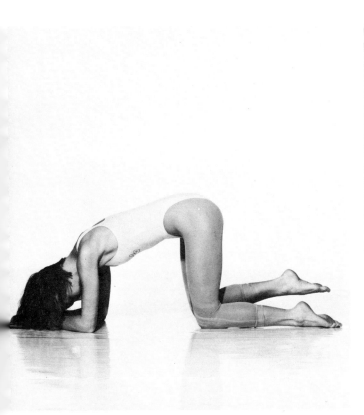
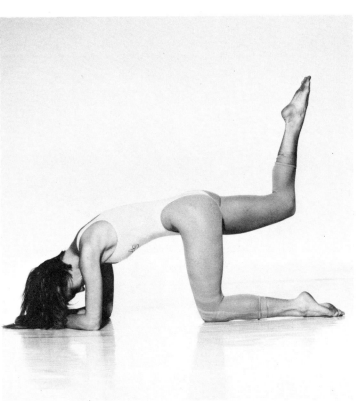

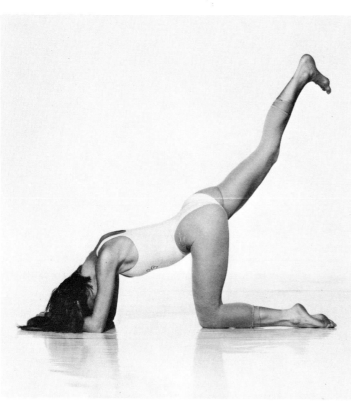

# 7 · DONKEY KICKS

1. Extend your right leg high up behind you. Flex your foot, squeeze your buttocks tight, and curl your pubic bone toward your navel to keep your back from arching.

2. Bend your flexed foot in toward your buttocks, keeping your knee lifted as high as possible.

3. Extend your leg again, lifting it higher.

Bend in and extend 16 times.

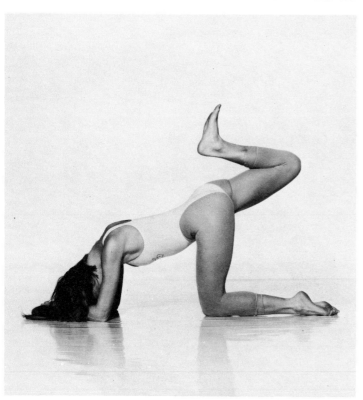

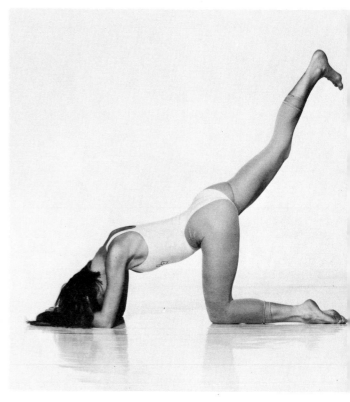

# $8 \cdot$ LEG EXTENSIONS

1. Point your toes and extend your right leg as high as possible. Squeeze the buttocks and lift the leg 8 times in very small movements. Then hold the leg high for 8 counts.

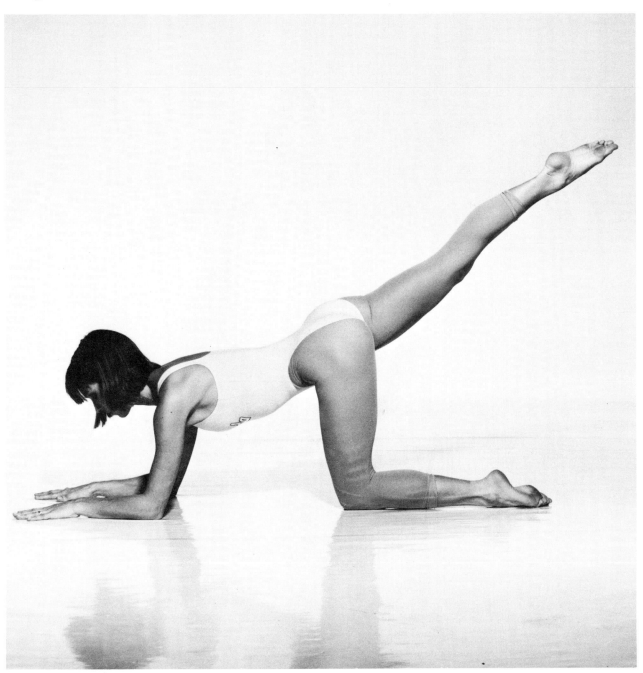

# 9 · TAILOR POSITION

1. Cross your right leg (the one you've been working) in front of your left leg.

2. Round down over your *left* knee. Relax and breathe. Feel the stretch in the right hip.

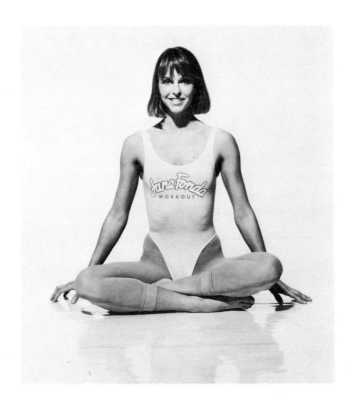

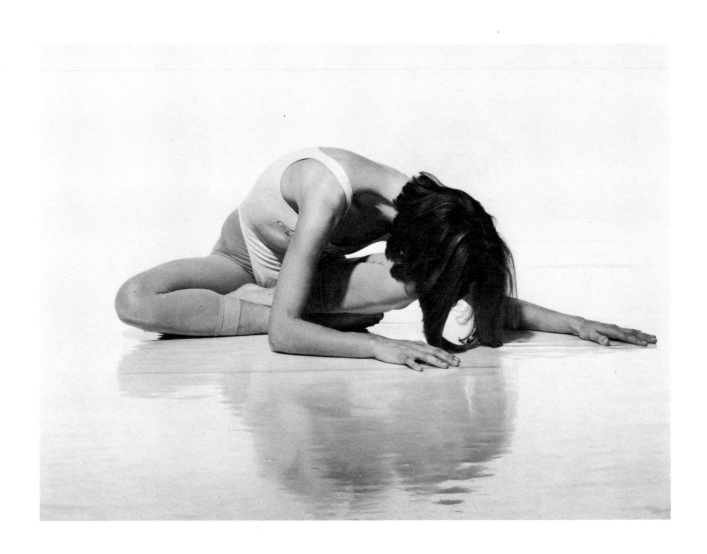

# 10 · TORSO STRETCH

Straighten up and wrap your left arm around your bent right knee and gently press the knee to your chest. Your left leg is bent, foot close to right hip, your back is straight, your right palm is flat on the floor behind your back. Look over your right shoulder and breathe deeply.

*Now we'll repeat the entire sequence of leg and hip exercises, starting with the Parallel Leg Lifts, working the left leg.*

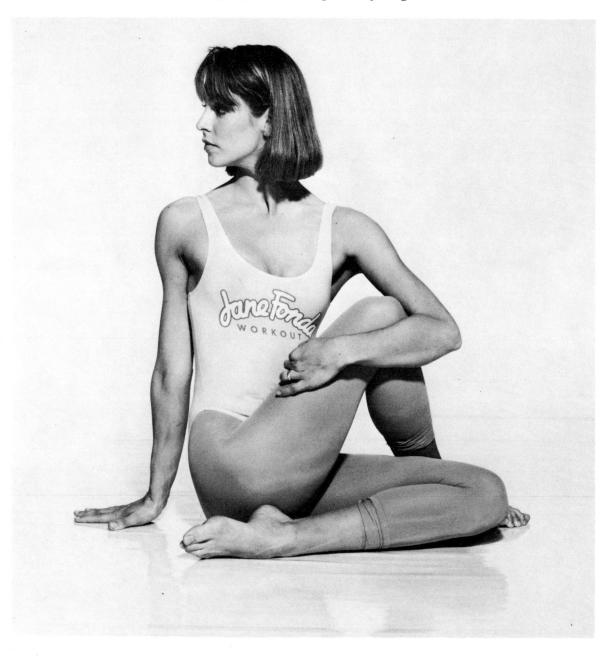

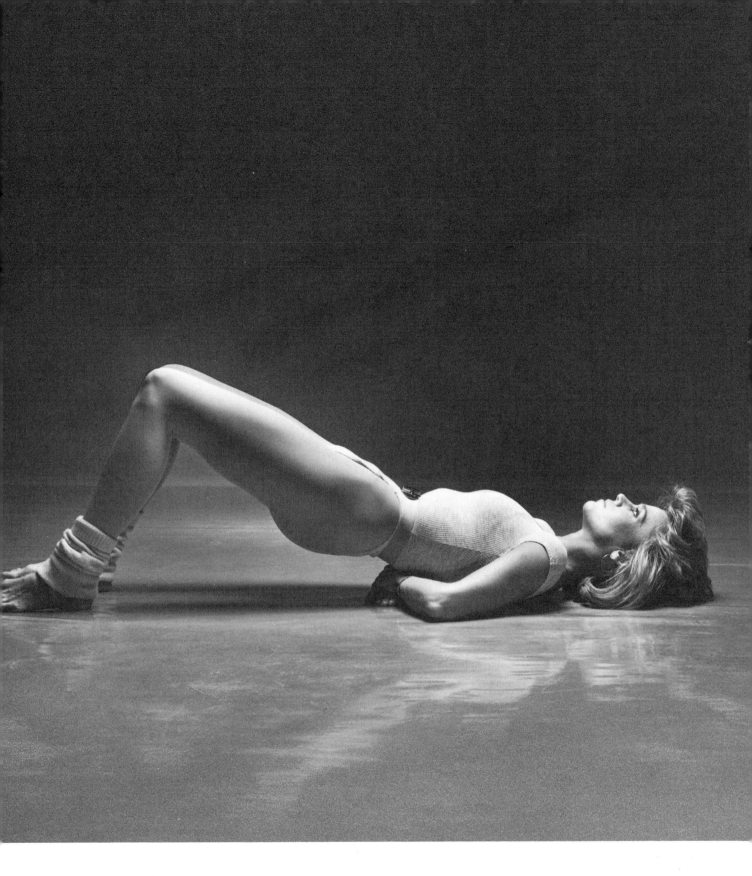

# Buttocks

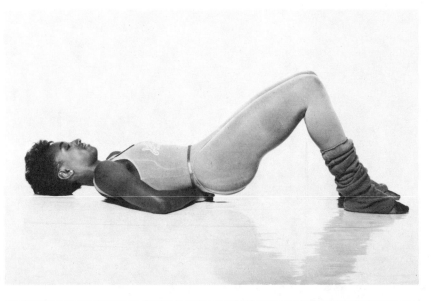

# 1 · PELVIC CURLS

These movements are very small but intense. Your hips may only move a few inches.

1. Lie on your back, feet and knees parallel, a little more than hip-distance apart. Place one hand on top of the other, palms down, directly beneath your lower back, which should touch your hands at all times.

2. Curl your pubic bone upward toward your navel, squeezing your buttock muscles as you do . . .

3. then relax these muscles a little.

Do steps 2 and 3 slowly 32 times and faster 24 times.

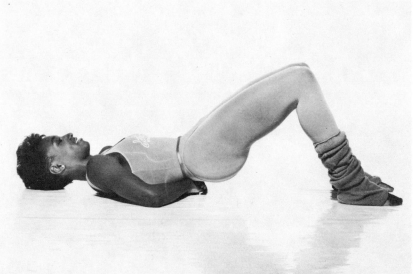

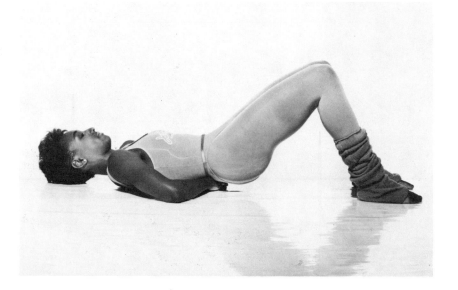

# 2 · KNEE PRESSES

1. Move your feet a little farther apart. With pubic bone curled upward, bring your knees apart . . .

2. and together, squeezing your buttock muscles even tighter as you bring knees together.

Steps 1 and 2 are done to 1 count. Do 24 counts slowly, then 24 counts faster, while keeping your buttocks tightly squeezed.

Resist the movement of your knees coming together. This should work your inner thigh as well as your buttocks. Think of bringing the upper part of your inner thighs, the part closest to the buttocks, together first.

*Do not let your back arch.*

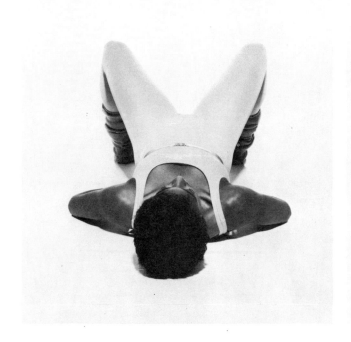 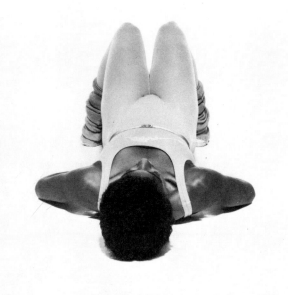

# 3 · BURN-OUT

1. Press your knees toward each other (they don't have to touch), then curl your buttocks upward and release them slightly 32 times.

Keep your lower back touching your hands. You should feel it deep inside the buttock muscles.

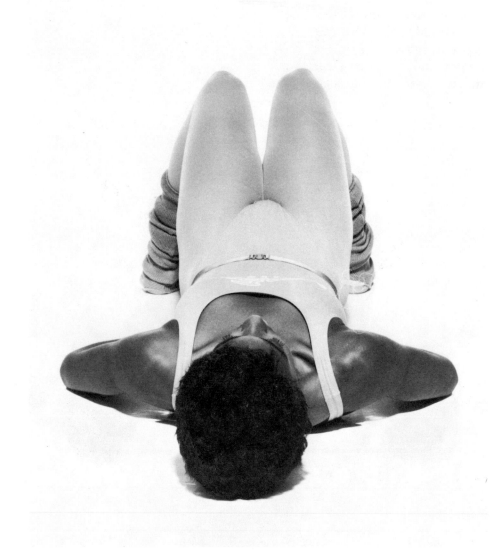

*Go right into the Cool-down without stopping.*

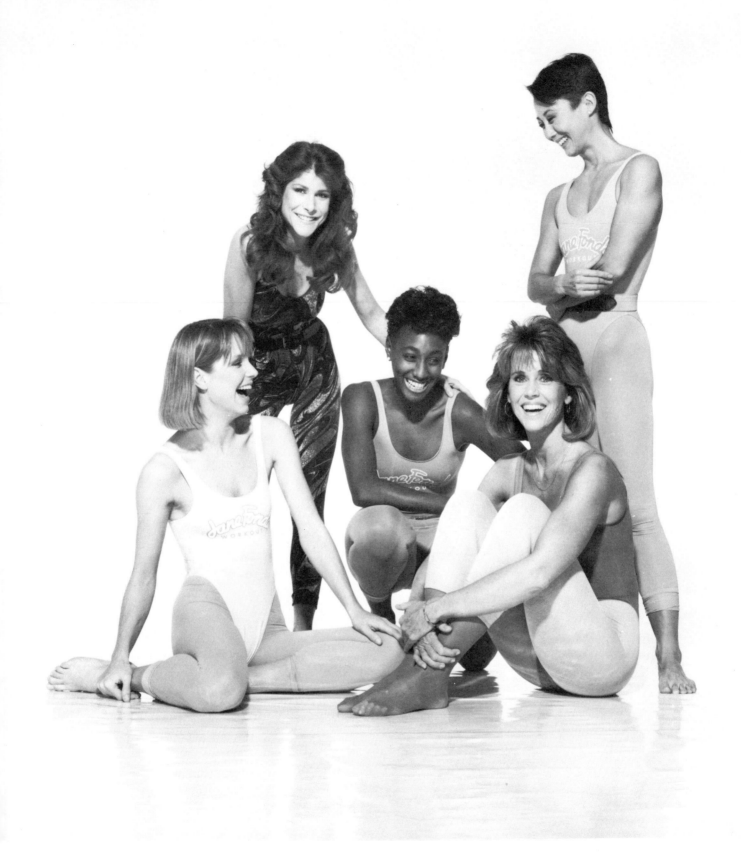

# Cool-down

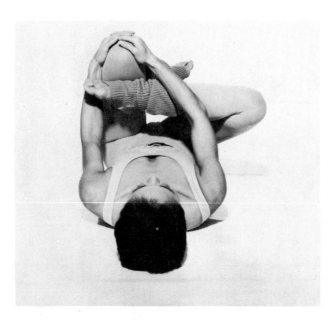

# 1 · HIP AND HAMSTRING STRETCH

1. Place your right ankle against your left knee and with your hands pull your left knee to your chest, stretching the right hip. Hold for 8 counts.

2. Place your left foot on the floor and stretch that right leg straight up, pressing it gently toward your chest with toes pointed . . .

3. then flexed.

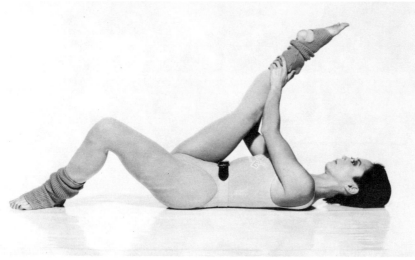

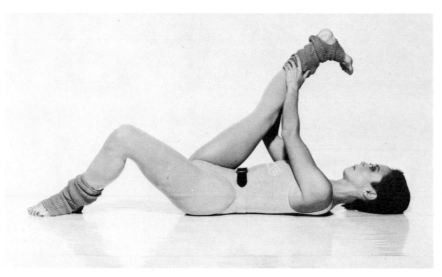

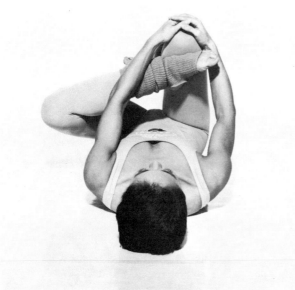

4. Place your left ankle against your right knee, and with your hands pull your right knee to your chest, stretching the left hip. Hold for 8 counts.

5. Place your right foot on the floor and stretch that left leg straight up, pressing it gently toward your chest with toes pointed . . .

6. then flexed.

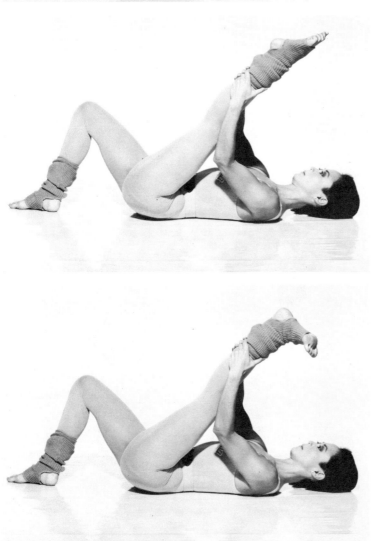

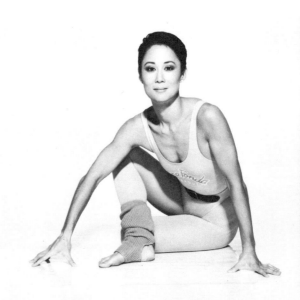

Roll up to a sitting position and bring one leg across the other. With foot flat on floor push off and come to a standing position with feet apart.

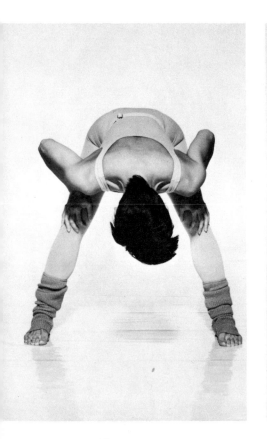

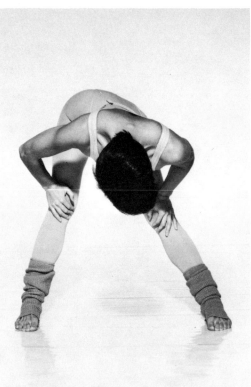

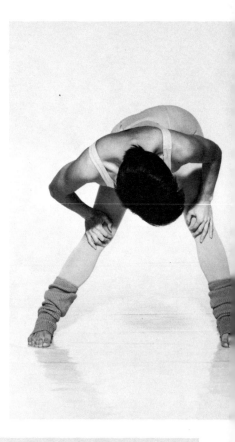

# 2 · GROIN STRETCH

1. Let your upper body drop down over your straight legs with hands on your thighs or knees.

2. Press your hips to the right . . .

3. and to the left.

Feel a stretch in the groin. Repeat once on each side, then bend your knees and roll up.

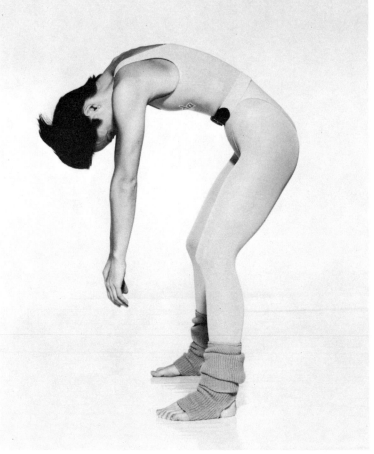

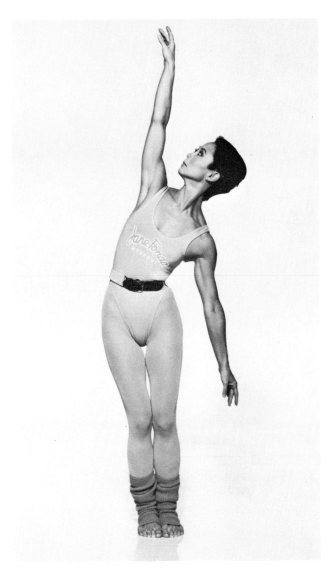
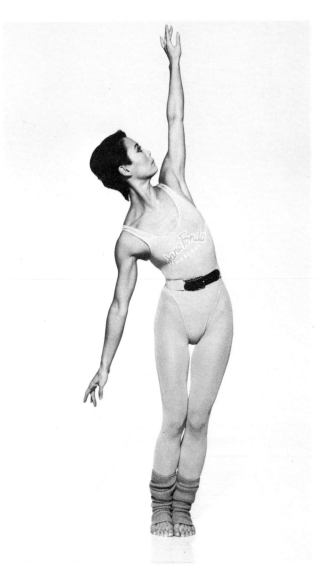

# 3 · SIDE STRETCH

1. Bring your feet together, knees bent. Reach up with your right arm and down with your left arm. Twist your torso slightly toward the raised arm. Look up toward the raised arm and feel a stretch up that side. Knees stay bent.

2. Repeat to the other side, reaching up with your left arm and down with your right arm. Look up toward your raised left arm and feel a stretch up that side. Knees stay bent.

**GOOD GOING! KEEP IT UP!**

# WORKOUT RESOURCES

## BOOKS

### Jane Fonda's Workout Book

My first book on health and fitness (now revised and replaced by my new Workout and Weight-Loss Program). Along with the basics of good nutrition and exercise, I present the original Workout—based on the Beginner's and Advanced exercises first offered at the Workout Studios. Available in both hard and soft cover.

### Women Coming of Age

My second book, which presents a complete nutrition and exercise program for midlife well-being. I address myself to women 35 to 65 years of age on virtually every aspect of concern in the middle years: the process of aging, the skin, middle-age spread, menopause, and taking care of the joints, the back, and the bones. The Prime Time Workout exercises are introduced here. Available in hard and soft cover. Written with Mignon McCarthy.

NOTE: *Women Coming of Age* is also available in an audio version, a 90-minute book on cassette.

### Jane Fonda's Workout Book for Pregnancy, Birth, and Recovery
by Femmy DeLyser

This book presents the unique pregnancy program created by Femmy DeLyser to guide women safely through the rapid physical changes involved in becoming a mother. It covers the entire year from conception to recovery and nursing, includes birthing skills and baby massage, and presents the special exercise program given at the Workout Studios for expectant and new mothers. Available in hard and soft cover.

## ALBUMS, AUDIOS, and VIDEOS

### 1. The New Workout

- *Jane Fonda's Workout Record—New and Improved (album)*
- *Jane Fonda's Workout—New and Improved* (audio cassette)
- *Jane Fonda's New Workout* (video cassette, Beta and VHS)

Excellent companions to this book, an updated album, audio cassette, and video of the basic Workout, Beginner's and Advanced, including an extended aerobics section. Special emphasis is given to exercising safely and with proper form. Both the album and audio cassette come complete with a manual of diagrams and instructions that make the exercises easy to follow. The Beginner's Workout on the album and audio cassette takes 30 minutes; on the video, 35 minutes. The Advanced Workout on the album and audio cassette takes 50 minutes; on the video, 55 minutes.

### 2. The Prime Time Workout

- *Jane Fonda's Prime Time Workout Record* (album)
- *Jane Fonda's Prime Time Workout* (audio cassette)
- *Jane Fonda's Prime Time Workout* (video cassette, Beta and VHS)

To complement the Prime Time Workout exercises introduced in *Women Coming of Age,* I've designed an album, audio cassette, and video. Each offers a 45-minute program designed especially for women and men in midlife and also for those who want a comprehensive exercise program but find the Beginner's and Advanced Workout from my first book too difficult. Prime Time is also excellent for anyone who does the regular Workout but simply wants a change of pace. With its emphasis on flexibility and proper form, Prime Time is especially good for those who haven't been exercising, who may be overweight, or who are suffering from back problems, arthritis, or injuries due to overuse.

3. *The Challenge Workout*

   • *Jane Fonda's Workout Challenge* (video cassette, Beta and VHS)

   For experienced exercisers, a vigorous 90-minute video cassette class. The Challenge is designed to build strength, to develop flexibility, and to increase endurance. Excellent for those who have been doing the Advanced Workout and feel ready to move on to a more strenuous class with 20 minutes of choreographed, highly energetic aerobics.

4. *The Stretch and Tone Workout (available Fall 1986)*

   • *Jane Fonda's Stretch and Tone Workout,* (video cassette, Beta and VHS)

   A program that concentrates on deep stretching and deep muscle toning. Excellent for developing greater flexibility and strength. Ideal for alternating with the other Workout programs.

5. *The Pregnancy, Birth, and Recovery Workout*

   • *Jane Fonda's Workout Record for Pregnancy, Birth, and Recovery* (album)
   • *Jane Fonda's Workout for Pregnancy, Birth, and Recovery* (audio cassette)
   • *Jane Fonda's Pregnancy, Birth, and Recovery Workout* (video cassette, Beta and VHS)

   Based on Femmy DeLyser's book, each of these—the album, audio cassette, and video—offers a complete 90-minute program led by Femmy and myself.

## Where to Find Workout Resources

The Workout books, albums, audio cassettes, and videos are available locally at all regular outlets. You may also order by mail. Write to:

The Workout, Inc.
P.O. Box 2957
Beverly Hills, CA 90213

# ILLUSTRATION CREDITS